The case for
PRECONCEPTION CARE
OF MEN AND WOMEN

The case for
PRECONCEPTION CARE
OF MEN AND WOMEN

Margaret Wynn and Arthur Wynn

A B ACADEMIC PUBLISHERS

Published in the UK by
AB Academic Publishers
PO Box 42
Bicester
Oxon OX6 7NW

© A B Academic Publishers 1991

British Library Cataloguing in Publication Data
Wynn, Margaret
  The case for preconception care of men and women.
  1. Man. Reproduction. Genetic factors
  I. Title II. Wynn, Arthur
  612.6

ISBN 0-907360-17-3

Phototypeset by David John Services Ltd, Berkshire
Printed in Great Britain

Contents

1. Care before conception and the outcome of pregnancy

Care before conception includes care by a couple of themselves and care of a couple by doctors and nurses. What is the evidence that a couple can do things before conception that may improve their chances of having a healthy baby? Does the health of a couple matter before conception? Does the health of a father really affect the outcome of pregnancy? What is meant by the 'health' of a couple? Are there hazards in everyday life which may prejudice a couple's chances of having a healthy baby? What is the evidence that there are periods of susceptibility of sperm and ova before and around the time of conception? The answers to these questions assume a greater importance when doctors or nurses advise disappointed couples who fail to conceive, have had a miscarriage or have had a stillborn baby, a baby that required intensive care or a baby with a handicap.

BIRTH-SPACING IS AN EXAMPLE OF PRECONCEPTION CARE

Is 'before' conception defined in months even years, in weeks or days or even hours before a conception takes place? One event which indisputably occurs before a conception is a preceding birth. The increase in infant mortality associated with too close birth-spacing is illustrated in Figure 1.1 based on American data. The British Births Survey 1970 showed that about 13 per cent of low birthweight and perinatal mortality was attributable to too close birth-spacing (Chamberlain et al., 1978). The increase in perinatal mortality is illustrated in Figure 1.2. Studies sponsored by the World Health Organization have estimated the infant deaths attributable to birth-spacing under 2 years in some 40 different countries which ranged from 5 to 40 per cent of all infant deaths with an average of about 18 per cent (Maine & McNamara, 1985).

The risk of low birthweight for the following baby also increases as the interval between births is reduced, as illustrated in Figure 1.3 for over one million births recorded in American official statistics. Growth of embryo and fetus is a result of cell replication and low birthweight is a consequence of a reduced rate of cell replication, except in those cases when late in pregnancy the baby is born too soon. If embryonic cell replication rate falls there is an increased risk of congenital malformations caused by what has been described as 'asynchronous differential growth' (Eckhert & Hurley, 1977). Too close birth-spacing increases the risk of congenital malformations as illustrated in

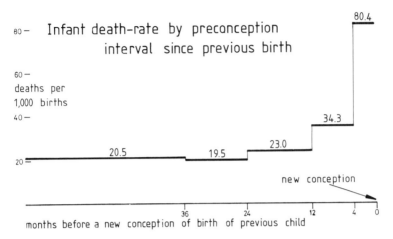

Figure 1.1. Kauai Survey, Territory of Hawaii 1953, 27,528 births.
Source: Yerushalmy *et al.*, 1956, Table II.

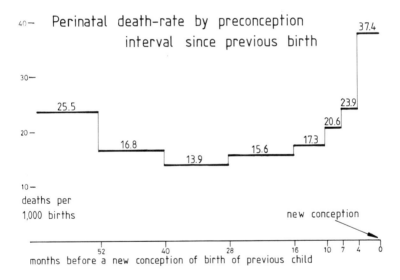

Figure 1.2. British Births Survey 1970, 10,336 births with interval recorded.
Source: Chamberlain *et al.*, 1978, Table 2.10.

Figure 1.4 for neural defects. In this Australian study by Field and Kerr (1981) there were 80 cases of anencephalus or meningomyelocele of which 29, or 36 per cent, were born less than one year after the previous birth, while only 4 or 5, or about 6 per cent, would have been expected if close birth-spacing had not increased risk. Too close birth-spacing can therefore produce a condition in the mother that results in a slow-down in cell replication very early in the next pregnancy.

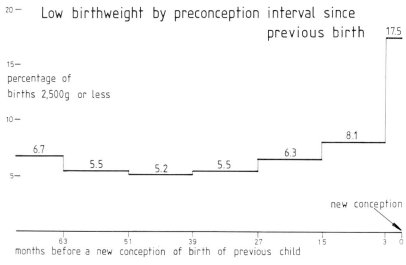

Figure 1.3. United States 1973–5, over one million births.
Source: US National Center for Health Statistics, 1978.

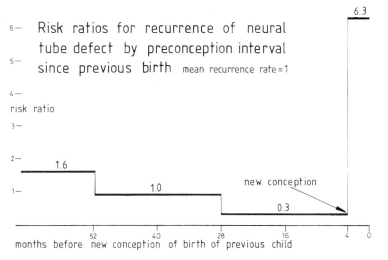

Figure 1.4. Australian study of anencephalus and meningomyelocele, 80 cases.
Source: Field & Kerr, 1981, Table 1.

In his introduction to a manual on prepregnancy care of women Chamberlain (1986) describes the two components of care: The larger is the appropriate and desirable knowledge for young people which is part of health education which is in turn part of education for living; the smaller component is medical and is concerned with identifiable problems meriting treatment. The knowledge that there is a desirable birth-spacing of 2 to 4 years and that birth-spacing under 2 years is unwise belongs to appropriate knowledge for all young people.

The most important conclusions in the present book are all such appropriate parts of health education rather than conclusions about the treatment of patients. Conclusions like the desirability of adequate birth-spacing are generally simple, but the supporting evidence necessary to convince doctors, nurses and parents is often far from simple; only world-wide studies sponsored by the World Health Organization have made it clear how serious the contribution of too close birth-spacing is to reproductive casualties and, indeed, years afterwards to small size and poor performance at school (Martin, 1978).

Some understanding of the concept of risk is a necessary part of the education of all young people and couples if they are to look after their own health. Close birth-spacing does not, of course, inevitably cause disaster but increases the risks. There is no certainty but only an increase in risks as birth-spacing is reduced as shown in Figures 1 to 4. Preconception care, and indeed most of preventive medicine, is concerned with reducing risks. The risks of an unfavourable pregnancy outcome cannot be reduced to zero but only ever to a level which is a best possible for a particular couple. It is noteworthy that satisfactory pregnancy spacing depends upon action by the couple themselves and the role of the health professional is that of conveying the knowledge that risks increase progressively as spacing is reduced below 2 years. Many parents of more than one child will tell you that they were told nothing by the health services about the importance of birth-spacing.

LOW BIRTHWEIGHT IS AN INDICATOR OF RISK

The appropriate knowledge for disappointed couples who fail to conceive, have miscarriages, stillborn, frail or handicapped children is more extensive than the knowledge appropriate for all young people. Such couples are concerned to prevent a repetition. The writers when visiting a neonatal intensive care unit met a young mother visiting her second low birthweight baby in an incubator. This young mother had been given no advice whatever between pregnancies on how to reduce the risk of a recurrence. The staff of the maternity hospital where both babies were born, general practitioner, community midwife or health visitor had all said nothing after the first pregnancy about timing of the second pregnancy or about the many other ways of reducing the risks of low birthweight discussed in the present book.

Too close birth-spacing is only one of many causes of slow-down of embryonic cell replication, low birthweight of embryonic origin and congenital malformation. The association of congenital malformation and low birthweight is general as illustrated from the statistics from England and Wales in Figure 1.5 for neural tube defects and Figure 1.6 for heart defects. The congenitally malformed heart has cells normal in size but generally reduced in number (Cheek *et al.*, 1966). Low birthweight has been reported to increase the risk

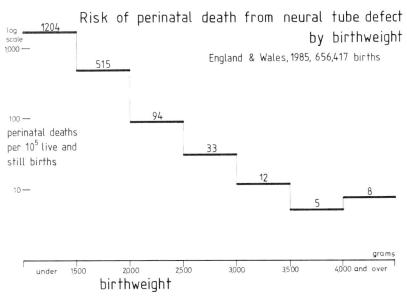

Figure 1.5. England and Wales 1985, 656,417 live births. Source: OPCS, 1988.

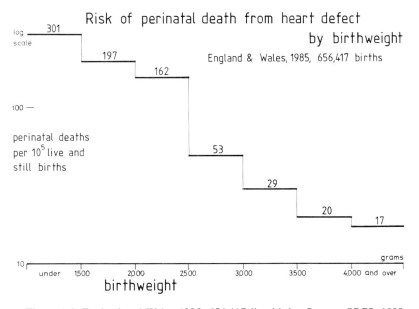

Figure 1.6. England and Wales 1985, 656,417 live births. Source: OPCS, 1988.

in the adult later in life of ischaemic heart disease and raised blood pressure (Barker & Osmund, 1986; Barker *et al.*, 1989; Whincup *et al.*, 1989).

The normal rate of cell replication during embryonic development is very much higher than later in pregnancy. Low birthweight matters most when it is associated with malformation and maldevelopment of early origin, at the time when cells are differentiating as well as dividing. The mass of the zygote after conception is about 4 micrograms but the foetus reaches 14-grams at the end of the first trimester. The mass has to double about 22 times between conception and the end of the first trimester, but the mass then only doubles 8 times until the end of pregnancy to reach 3,500g. In fact the zygote before first cleavage is more than 1,000 times larger than the average cell of the foetus at the end of the first trimester. The zygote requires at least another 10 doublings to reduce the cell size so that total doublings during the first trimester are more than 32 without allowing for cell death. Early cell replication is part of a genetically determined program and if part of the program is omitted it cannot be reinstated later, any more than it is possible for an actor to reinstate lines of a play in the third Act that he accidentally omitted from the first. Most congenital malformations may be regarded as the result of omissions of part of the genetic program of cell replication. The risk of such omissions increases if the rate of cell replication slows down below the programmed rate.

Congenital malformations and low birthweight may be caused by insults during early pregnancy to the developing embryo and they may also be caused by insults to germ cells before conception. It may then be asked whether too

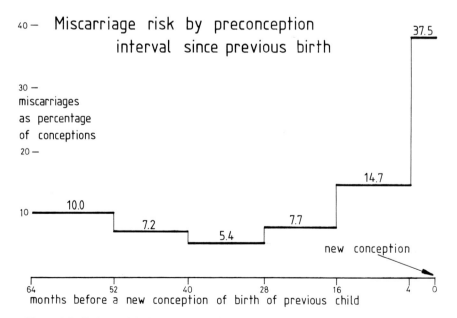

Figure 1.7. Turkey, 18,015 pregnancies. Source: Sümbüloglu *et al.*, 1976, Table 3.D.6.

close birth-spacing damages the female germ cell or ovum before conception. The answer to this question is to be found by studying miscarriage, particularly early miscarriage which is the commonest form of pregnancy failure. The risk of miscarriage in a second pregnancy increases as the birth interval falls below 2 years as illustrated in Figure 1.7 based on a study sponsored by WHO of pregnancies in Ankara, Turkey (Omran & Standley, 1976). Several studies have shown that more than one half all miscarried embryos have chromosomal abnormalities. Thus a study at the University of British Columbia of 228 embryos aborted found that 129 or 57 per cent, had chromosomal abnormalities (Poland *et al.*, 1981). What then is the origin of these chromosomal abnormalities? Such abnormalities are defects in the genome, and therefore must have their origin before or sometimes around conception. The origin of defects in female germ cell or ovum is discussed further in Chapter Two and in male germ cell or sperm in Chapter Three.

ONE-GENERATION GENETIC DISEASE

Concern at the apparently growing number of causes of damage to germ cells in our complex urban world persuaded leading countries to establish 'environmental mutagen societies' about 1960. A report of the European society defined a 'mutation' very broadly as 'an alteration in the genetic apparatus of an organism' (European Environmental Mutagen Society, 1978). More than half of all early miscarriages are by this definition caused by mutations. Furthermore by this definition too close birth-spacing causes mutation in maternal cells. The international body of national environmental mutagen societies published a report on estimation of the diseases caused by new mutations in man and said (ICPEMC, 1983):

> 'Mutagenic agents may cause genetic damage in any cell of the body. If the damage occurs in somatic cells it may lead to cancer, or other degenerative diseases in the exposed individual. In a somatic cell of a foetus such genetic damage may result in congenital abnormality. However, if the damage occurs in a germ cell, it may be transmitted to the next or later generations where it may cause disease.'

This quotation refers to the foetus and includes the early or embryonic period of two months after conception when the genetic apparatus of the dividing and differentiating somatic cells of the embryo is particularly susceptible to damage.

Because the cause of some disorder is environmental the origin is not necessarily postconceptional. An environmental factor may cause a mutation in a germ cell. Such a mutation is an event before conception. Research over many years has shown that there are numerous environmental causes of mutation including radiation and many chemicals, and rates of mutation are modulated by acidity, alkalinity, temperature, intracellular concentrations of hormones and nutrients and viral diseases. Because the cause of some disorder is 'genetic' it is not necessarily inherited from grandparents because it may be mutational in origin. A disorder that is inherited may not be inherited from grandparents or more distant ancestors but only from parents whose germ cells acquired a mutation. Such a disorder may be called a one-generation genetic disease.

Some serious disorders are inherited from parents but are not compatible with reproduction and sufferers have no descendants yet the disease persists in the general population. Down's syndrome is such a disorder. Only 24 women with Down's syndrome have been reported to have had a child, and no men with Down's syndrome to have done so (Jagiello, 1981). Down's syndrome is genetic and inherited; sufferers have an extra chromosome 21. But Down's syndrome is not inherited from grandparents except in perhaps 5 per cent of cases where there is a predisposing mosaicism or a translocation, which may be acquired from grandparents. Down's syndrome is an example of a one-generation genetic disease caused by mutations in parental germ cells. The prevalence of Down's syndrome in the community is almost wholly maintained by new mutations in parental germ cells at times discussed in later chapters. A report on estimation of diseases caused by new mutations in man by ICPEMC (1983) concluded:

'Thus, in man mutation must be considered essentially harmful. In addition, the harmfulness of mutation can be seen from the fact that a variety of diseases depends on repeated mutation for their continued presence in the population.'

'Thus natural selection tends to eliminate the genes or chromosome changes concerned from the population and the incidence of the conditions depends upon a balance between selection, tending to decrease the incidence, and new mutations, tending to increase it. Thus, an increase in the rate of mutation will raise the incidence'.

The fertility of sufferers from Down's syndrome is virtually zero so that the incidence is proportional to the rate of mutation. The report refers to epilepsy, schizophrenia, many kinds of congenital malformation, diabetes and many other disorders as partly genetic in origin with a depressed fertility of sufferers and with a prevalence partly maintained by new mutations.

NEW MUTATIONS ARE A CAUSE OF HANDICAP

The decline in infant and perinatal mortality over the last half century has not been matched by a decline in birth defects. The US Centers for Disease Control (1989) say that the USA will not reach its national target for lowering infant mortality because birth defects are not falling. The prevention of undesirable mutations is an essential part of programs aimed at preventing birth defects and handicap. Undesirable mutations are a cause not only of physical defects which are apparent at birth but also of defects with no obvious dysmorphology. Mutations are, in particular, responsible for a range of defects of the central nervous system which are among the most serious human burdens. Studies in Britain, Sweden, Germany and elsewhere have shown that psychiatric patients are subfertile (Slater *et al.*, 1971; Larsen & Nyman, 1973). The lower marriage rate and the lower fertility of those who marry reduces fertility to approximately one half that of the general population, so that prevalence would fall by about 50 per cent per generation if it depended only on the reproduction of psychiatric patients and upon them all having abnormal children. However the very great majority of psychiatric patients have normal parents and the prevalence of psychiatric disorders is not falling.

The fragile-X syndrome is the commonest cause of mental subnormality in men after Down's syndrome (Moser, 1985). Fragile sites or break-points in chromosomes, of which some 30 or 40 including the fragile-X site have been identified, are associated with an increased risk of miscarriage and stillbirth (Hecht & Hecht, 1984). The clinical significance otherwise of most fragile sites is not known execpt for the site on the X-chromosome at Xq27 associated with mental subnormality in the male. Sutherland, who was a pioneer in the discovery of the fragile-X syndrome, studied 104 cases from 95 unrelated families and concluded that the syndrome was the result of new mutations (Mulley & Sutherland, 1983). Mothers can be carriers of the fragile-X syndrome, but are only slightly affected if affected at all, and can transmit the mutation from a grandfather. Sutherland found that the sufferers were almost all infertile, but the syndrome is constantly regenerated from mutations in father, mother, grandfather and exceptionally in more remote forebears (Winter, 1987). The fragile-X syndrome is an exception to a general association of mental subnormality and small size.

Epilepsy is another example of a disease which is partly caused by one-generational genetic inheritance. A study of 274 pairs of identical twins found that when one twin had epilepsy so had the other in 57 per cent of cases, while in 570 pairs of non-identical twins the concordance was only 11 per cent as shown in Table 1.1 (Tsuboi & Endo, 1977). These twin studies suggest that the genetic contribution to the prevalence of epilepsy is around 50 per cent. However averaging the results of 7 studies of 6,822 epileptic parents the risk of a child being epileptic if only one parent was epileptic was only 3.5 per cent as shown in Table 1.2 (Janz *et al.*, 1982). A study from Montreal found that young men and women with epilepsy particularly young men, have lower marriage rates than normal and only about half the average number of

TABLE 1.1

TWIN STUDIES OF EPILEPSY

	one epileptic	both epileptic	concordance per cent
monozygotic twins	119	155	57
dizygotic twins	509	61	11

Source: Tsuboi & Endo, 1977; summary of 17 series, 844 sets of twins

children (Dansky *et al.*, 1980). Combining the effects of lower fertility and risk of inheritance from an epileptic parent it is found that less than 2 per cent of epileptics have epileptic parents. Ninety-eight per cent of epileptics are born to parents with no family history of epilepsy. Epilepsy is continually dying out but is continually regenerated partly by new mutations in parental germ cells and partly by insults after conception and after birth. Low birthweight and small head circumference are both risk factors for many brain disorders including epilepsy. A series of 265 patients with congenital cerebral palsy in a Danish study included 81 who had single convulsions or epilepsy. Twenty-six per cent of the epileptic patients had birthweights under 2,500g (Glenting, 1970).

TABLE 1.2

CHILDREN WITH ONE EPILEPTIC PARENT WHO HAVE EPILEPSY

number of couples (one epileptic):	6,822
number of their children:	5,357
number of children with epilepsy:	188 or 3.5 per cent

Source: Janz *et al.*, 1982; summary of 7 studies

Smaller size is not necessarily evidence of lower intelligence. The Shire horse is not more intelligent than the Shetland pony, and elephants are not more intelligent than people. If small size is part of normal genetic programming it has no such direct connection with mental performance. If however, small size is a consequence of slow-down in embryonic growth there is an increased risk of educational subnormality. Studies of American children in the 1940s reported 'an unexpectedly high relation between intelligence quotients and stature' (Boas, 1941). A study of children attending English special schools for the educationally subnormal reported that these children were also physically backward with average heights and weights substantially below the average (Parry-Jones & Murray, 1958). There was a debate on whether the unusually small children at these special schools were 'an expression of man's genetic variability' or were small because of inadequacy of the home environment. These are not the only two alternatives.

Growth retardation or small size may begin with mutation in the germ cells of mother or father as well as in remote ancestors, or at any time after conception during the development of the zygote or embryo. Small size at birth may or may not be wholly or partially corrected by subsequent catch-up. But if the newborn is small for gestational age and there is no subsequent catch-up there is cause for concern. There is a risk of educational subnormality if head circumference at birth is below the 10th percentile and remains below the 10th percentile in early childhood (Dunn *et al.*, 1986)

Educational subnormality has many postnatal causes, is difficult to measure and however measured has a continuous scale extending from normality to

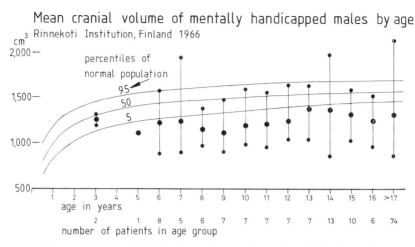

Figure 1.8. Finland, 359 patients. Source: Iivanainen, 1974, Figure 9.

extreme forms of handicap. The cases of only slight or moderate degrees of mental handicap often of postnatal origin are numerically and therefore socially of greater importance than the small number of serious cases requiring long-term hospital care. However, the origin of much mental handicap can be seen more clearly by study of the more serious cases. There is just one physical characteristic that the majority of the severely mentally subnormal have in common. They are very little people and in particular have small heads. The cranial volumes of 358 severely subnormal patients at the Rinnekoti Institute in Finland are shown in Figure 1.8 (Iivanainen, 1974). The cranial volumes of 207 patients were below the 5th percentile, that is 74 per cent of the total, while only 10 patients had cranial volumes above the 95th percentile. About 95 per cent of the 358 patients were below the 50th percentile of height for age and 180 or over one half were below the 2.5 percentile. At some stage in their development these little people had suffered a slow-down in cell replication. In 18 per cent of cases there was evidence of postnatal trauma or infection and in a further 12 per cent of cases there was evidence of trauma or hypoxia or other perinatal cause of the handicap. In 69 per cent of cases there was some malformation of the skull, as well as small skull volume, a combination likely to have its origin in early pregnancy or earlier still. Growth retardation of the head is more closely associated with neurological deficits than growth retardation of the rest of the body as commonsense would anticipate (Gross *et al.*, 1978; Nelson & Deutschberger, 1970). The US Collaborative Perinatal Study provided information on the children found to be neurologically abnormal at one year of age on 31,240 children. The risk of neurological abnormality for infants with birthweights under 2,500g was 3.35 times that of the infants who had higher birthweights (Niswander & Gordon, 1972).

SUSCEPTIBILITY OF GERM-CELL STAGES

If an important part of all handicap has its origin very early in pregnancy the only hope of primary prevention must depend upon intervention before conception. If, furthermore, embryonic development is prejudiced by mutations before conception then preconception care is also indicated. The period before conception when germ cells are particularly susceptible to mutagens does however need to be defined. In animals the risk of some particular insults causing a subsequent pregnancy failure by damaging germ cells has been reported to increase during the prepregnancy period by a 1,000 times or more (Adler, 1982a). There are periods of heightened susceptibility to mutagens extending forward into the embryonic period and backward into the period of maturation of germ cells. These periods of heightened susceptibility differ for different mutagenic agents, for different types of mutation, and for men and women (Lyon, 1988).

In 1981 Mary Lyon of the Medical Research Council, Radiobiology Unit, Harwell presented a paper to the International Commission entitled *Sensitivity of various germ-cell stages to environmental mutagens*. Among the conclusions the paper said:

'In instances in which exposure is not continuous but occasional it may be possible to remove a large part of the genetic hazard by avoiding conception for a few months after exposure. Such cases might include accidental exposure, or some types of medical treatment.'

This was among the first papers to underline the importance of the preconception period for the prevention of mutations and genetic damage.

The final report of the International Commission under the Chairmanship of Mary Lyon concluded (ICPEMC, 1983):

'It may be particularly important to know the risk to maturing stages of germ cells, since it may be possible to avoid the genetic harm done to these stages, if the accidentally exposed individuals refrain from conception for 3 months.'

The period of heightened susceptibility for women is discussed in Chapter Two and for men in Chapter Three. In both these chapters the causes of damage to germ cells and embryo are chosen for the light that they throw on these susceptible periods rather than for their common occurrence. Counselling to reduce the risk of handing on recessive disorders to the next generation is outside the scope of this book. Evidence is, however, introduced aimed at reducing genetic harm caused by new mutations.

2. Susceptible periods in women

SUSCEPTIBILITY TO MUTATION AROUND OVULATION

There is a period immediately around ovulation when the maturing ovum is particularly easily damaged by many kinds of environmental hazard. Work sponsored by the US Atomic Energy Commission at the Oak Ridge National Laboratory showed that mice were highly sensitive to radiation during the 8.5 hours before mating which coincides with ovulation. Liane Russell (1956) wrote:

> 'Females irradiated 8.5 hours before fertilization produced only about one sixtieth as many living embryos as those irradiated at any stage 16 hours to $4\frac{1}{2}$ days before fertilization...'

In another paper the Russells wrote that a 70-fold increase in sensitivity occurs between 11.30 a.m. and 7 p.m. on the day preceding ovulation (Russell & Russell, 1956). These studies showed that the deaths of mice ova caused by radiation before ovulation were associated with damage to chromosomes. The results of animal experiments provide warnings that need when possible to be confirmed, but warnings that are to be taken seriously until shown to be wrong. The more species of animal to which some generalization applies the stronger is the hypothesis it generates for humans. The increase in susceptibility to environmental hazards during preovulatory maturation is shared by all mammals that have so far been the subject of experiment including other primates, but with differences between species in the length of the period of susceptibility.

The Russells' experiments were only concerned with the effects of radiation. A colleague of the Russells found that the susceptibility to chemicals also increased during the period before mating and around ovulation, and Figure 2.1 is based on his research (Generoso, 1969). Female mice were divided into 4 groups and were each given a dose of a mutagen at different times before ovulation. In the fourth group, dosed with the mutagenic chemical between 12 hours and 5 days before ovulation, it is seen that over 80 per cent of ova suffered mutations which were lethal, that is the embryo resulting from fertilization was dead or unable to survive for long. In contrast, it is seen that only 10 per cent had lethal mutations if the female mice were dosed with the mutagens from 15 to 20 days before ovulation. Fig 2.1 suggests that the shorter the interval between exposure to some hazard and ovulation, the greater the risk to the outcome of pregnancy. When thinking of humans, the timing is different from animals, but the principle is the same.

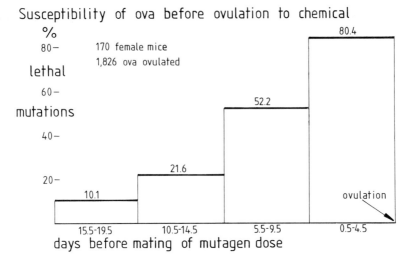

Figure 2.1. Dominant lethal mutations in female mice. Source: Generoso, 1969, Table 2.

Chemicals, unlike radiation, produce a somewhat blurred picture of the period of susceptibility around ovulation because they take time to reach and affect the ovum and usually disappear quite slowly over hours or days. Pulses of radiation show the quite rapid changes in susceptibility more clearly. The beginning of preovulatory maturation is marked by a rapid and substantial rise in the release of two pituitary hormones, follicle stimulating hormone (FSH) and luteinizing hormone (LH). The peak of LH release is shown in Figure 2.2. using data showing the radio-sensitivity of the ova of Chinese hamsters

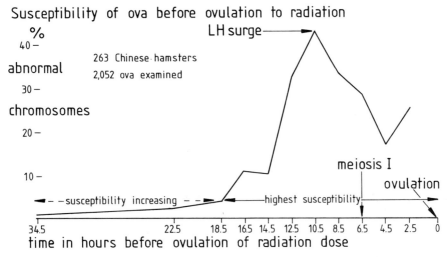

Figure 2.2. Chromosomal mutations around meiosis 1. Sources: Mikamo, 1982 Figure 2. Reprinted by permission of S. Karger AG, Basel. Wynn & Wynn 1988a, Figure 5.

from a study by Mikamo (1982) of Asahikawa Medical College. A pulse of radiation was given at 15 different times to separate groups of animals during the 84 hours before ovulation. The percentage of chromosomal abnormalities was recorded in ova recovered about 5 hours following ovulation at metaphase II without mating. Only animals maintaining a regular oestrous cycle were used. The peak of chromosomal aberrations caused by radiation is seen to coincide with exposure to a dose of radiation around the peak of the LH surge, about 10 hours before ovulation. During these 10 hours Mikamo's hamsters showed an increase in susceptibility to radiation of about 60 times. This is the same increase in susceptibility that the Russells reported in 1956. The time from the LH surge until ovulation includes meiosis I and the early preparatory stages of meiosis II. Not only mammals but some invertebrates have been shown to share this increased susceptibility to insult during the two stages of meiosis. In the male meiosis is also a time of high susceptibility to environmental hazards.

In Figure 2.2 the effect of radiation on the ova of non-mated female hamsters is shown. In later experiments reported in the same paper Mikamo and his team studied the numbers of embryos surviving 18.5. days, instead of 5 hours, after ovulation and mating, using the same doses of radiation at the same times before ovulation. Mikamo found the same period of high susceptibility in mated animals coinciding with ovulatory maturation, but found more deaths of embryos or 'dominant lethal mutations' than they expected from the chromosomal abnormalities measured in the previous experiments, particularly for the doses of radiation during the 8 hours before ovulation. Chromosomal abnormalities are generally lethal. It appeared that some of the effects of radiation took more than a few hours to become apparent. These further experiments emphasized that the high susceptibility persists through the whole period from LH surge until meiosis II.

SUSCEPTIBILITY TO MUTATION AROUND CONCEPTION

Meiosis II is completed in humans after a sperm enters the ovum. The chromosomal abnormalities reported in these experiments were 'new mutations' caused by radiation, following the definitions in Chapter One. The story is taken a step further in Figure 2.3 based on another study by Generoso which begins where Mikamo left off (Generoso *et al.*, 1987). The high susceptibility to poisons in mice is seen in Figure 2.3 to continue after mating. Generoso commented that it was at one time generally believed that chemicals and radiation only produce congenital abnormalities in surviving embryos much later after implantation of the ovum in the uterus when the embryo is actually producing the abnormal organs and limbs. 'This long-standing belief' said Generoso, was obviously wrong because he and his colleagues had succeeded in producing 'remarkable increases in the incidence of congenital abnormalities

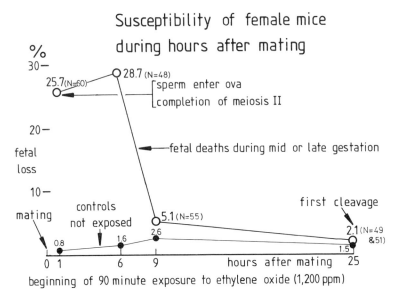

Figure 2.3. Fetal malformations and death from exposure to mutagens after mating.
Source: Generoso *et al.*, 1987, Figure 1..

and death of foetuses' by exposure to a mutagen only 1 hour or 6 hours after mating and not later in the embryonic period. At the time when Generoso exposed his mice to chemicals the fertilized ova were still only single cells. The organs and limbs did not yet exist except in the genetic code. Generoso suggests that damage by mutagens at this time is genetic damage, or in other words new mutations, causing the subsequent foetal loss. Mutations continue indeed to happen for a time after fertilization. Generoso in the experiments illustrated in Figure 2.3 used ethylene oxide as the mutagen. Ethylene oxide is an important industrial chemical used in the production of ethylene glycol, antifreeze for motor vehicles, and acrylic ester fibres. It is also used as a fumigant for foodstuffs, textiles and in the sterilization of surgical instruments. The interval between mating Generoso's mice and sperm entering ova is shown as only one hour. The mice were in 4 groups, the first given ethylene oxide an hour after mating the fourth around first cleavage. In women the interval may be 24 hours or even longer, and the time to first cleavage when the fertilized ovum divides for the first time may be 2 or 3 days. In Generoso's experiments exposure 1 or 6 hours after fertilization greatly increased the number of late foetal deaths as shown in Figure 2.3, but losses were much lower for exposure beginning 9 hours after fertilization and were not different from controls for exposure beginning 25 hours afterwards. These studies were repeated by the same team using three other chemical mutagens all of which produced developmental abnormalities following exposure of early zygotes. Two of the mutagens also produced high losses of conceptuses in all postmating stages up to implantation and later (Generoso *et al.*, 1988; Katoh *et al.*,

1989). A dilute solution of alcohol fed to female mice during this susceptible period around and immediately after mating has been shown by Kaufman in Cambridge (1983) to cause chromosomal abnormalities.

How long then, is the period of highest susceptibility in women? Figure 2.4. is an attempt to put the evidence together in a simplified picture of the susceptibility of women around ovulation. A safety factor is added at each end of the period. The time from ovulation to first cleavage, that is to completion of the first cell division to produce a 2-cell embryo, is normally about 1½ days (McLaren, 1982). This time can, however, be longer, particularly because the time between ovulation and fertilization may be longer. The time from ovulation to first cleavage is therefore shown conservatively as 2½ days. In women the time between the peak of the LH surge and ovulation is reported to be 30 to 36 hours (Edwards & Steptoe, 1975). In the interests of caution 36 hours is used in Figure 2.4. Assuming the human time-scale prior to ovulation is 3.3 times longer than that of the Chinese hamster the period of highest susceptibility of women would be as long as 60 hours prior to ovulation. The beginning of the period of highest susceptibility in Figure 2.4 is shown as 3 days, counting backwards from ovulation and allowing for some variation in the speed of events. Counting forwards from ovulation it is seen that the susceptibility is already decreasing before the first cleavage. It is therefore suggested that the whole period of highest susceptibility in Figure 2.4 lasts about 4½ days. The time of ovulation is usually about mid-cycle, or about 14 days after the first day of menses in a 28-day cycle. The length of cycle

Women's susceptibility around ovulation

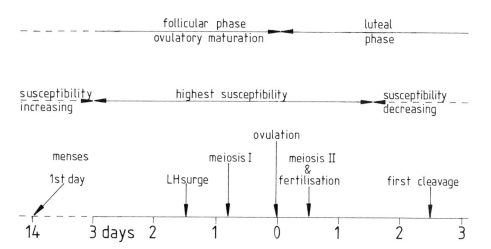

Figure 2.4. Time-table of susceptibility in women.

varies from under 25 days to over 35 days and the post-ovulatory part of the cycle varies between about 10 and 14 days.

A report on the animal testing of chemicals for mutagenicity proposed that initial testing should be restricted to the period around meiosis I and post-meiotic stages as no chemical has ever been shown to induce mutations which fails to do so during these active stages of meiosis (Epstein & Röhrborn, 1970). Furthermore chemicals that induce mutations during these meiotic stages may not produce any evidence of mutagenicity at other times at comparable doses. This report was, however, only concerned with dominant lethal testing and chromosomal abnormalities and to the exposure of mainly male animals to chemical mutagens. This kind of testing does not identify chemicals producing only gene mutations or deletions and can therefore only provide positive evidence of mutagenicity and can never show that a chemical is not mutagenic.

Mikamo counted lethal mutations but did not study mutations in survivors. Nomura (1982) of the Institute for Cancer Research, Osaka University, used both X-rays and a chemical mutagen, urethane, on both male and female mice before mating and studied congenital malformations and tumours in survivors. Urethane is a potent chemical mutagen but nevertheless does not cause dominant lethal mutations or chromosomal abnormalities. Examination of 5,830 embryos by Nomura revealed no significant increase of dominant lethal mutations following dosing of a parent with urethane. X-rays on the contrary produced dominant lethal mutations as expected. Most malformations and tumours are, however, caused by gene mutations not by visible chromosomal abnormalities and urethane given to male or female mice before mating was very effective in producing malformations as shown in Figure 2.5 and tumours as shown in Figure 2.6. In one series of Nomura's experiments malformations were recorded in 19-day old foetuses, as shown in Figure 2.5., and in a second series in 7-day old offspring. The rate of malformations fell by 50 per cent between 19 day old foetuses and 7 day old pups because of the high mortality shortly after birth. At 7 days there were more than 10 times as many malformed pups as in controls. One of the less lethal malformations, open eyelid, was shown to be heritable. The tumours were diagnosed in offspring at 8 months of age and were found to be heritable in experiments confined to the male line as far as the F_3 generation with a dominant pattern of inheritance and about 40 per cent penetrance. The strain of animals used may have had a particular susceptibility to tumour initiation. It is apparent, however, from these experiments that tumours in offspring can be produced by exposure of the parental germ line to mutagens before fertilization. The females were irradiated or dosed with urethane in what was described as the 'late follicular stage' which covered the 14 days before ovulation. As there are profound changes in female susceptibility during these 14 days Nomura's studies do not help in the detailed description of the susceptible period.

While the highest susceptibility in women may only last about 4½ days as suggested in Figure 2.4 animal experiments show that susceptibility, although at a lower level, increases from the beginning of the cycle, which in women is 14 days before ovulation and furthermore that susceptibility particularly to single gene mutations begins to increase earlier still as long as 40 days before mating in the mouse, equivalent to about 100 days in women (Russell, 1977).

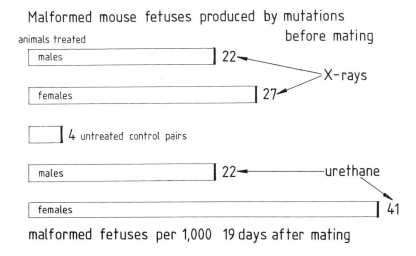

Figure 2.5. Malformations in 19-day fetuses. Mice treated with X-rays; males 2,201; females 942. Mice treated with urethane: males 3,400; females 1,262; controls 1,026. Sources: Nomura, 1982, Figure 2, Table 1. Reprinted by permission of Nature, Macmillan Magazines Ltd; Wynn & Wynn, 1989.

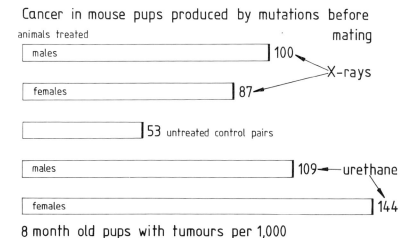

Figure 2.6. Cancer in 8-month pups. Mice treated with X rays: males 1,529; females 1,155. Mice treated with urethane: males 1,254; females 1,735; controls 548. Sources: Nomura, 1982, Figure 3; Wynn & Wynn, 1989.

Russell in one series of experiments examined 258,663 mouse pups for 7 specific mutations following irradiation of the dams with 50 rads at a rate of 50 rads/min. No mutations were recorded for 92,059 pups with an interval between irradiation of their dams and mating greater than 42 days. There were 7 mutations in 71,070 pups following irradiation 21 to 42 days before mating. Animal studies suggest that the dormant mammalian female germ line may be insensitive to the action of most mutagens until a few weeks before ovulation when the period of increased susceptibility begins (Oakberg, 1979). Does the comparative insensitivity of dormant germ cells apply to women?

Susceptibility in women must build up to the high level around ovulation, but there is no direct evidence as to how long this takes. The beginning of susceptibility 100 days before ovulation is a cautious estimate based on the animal experiments. Cox and Lyon (1975), of the Radiobiology Unit at Harwell, discussing their experiments on guinea pigs and hamsters, said that it would be imprudent to assume that no mutations could be induced by radiation in the dormant, or immature oocyte, and they added that it is reasonable to assume only that it is more difficult to cause mutations in the dormant human oocyte than in the mature oocyte. They also suggested that the susceptibility of the human oocyte during the period prior to ovulation may not be very different from that found in experimental mammals. This is a cautious assumption for couples and those who advise them.

SUSCEPTIBLE PERIODS FOR THE ORIGIN OF DOWN'S SYNDROME

The importance of susceptible periods may be shown by examining the origins of a particular genetic disease caused by chromosomal abnormality, namely Down's syndrome. The knowledge of when Down's syndrome originates is part of the knowledge needed for its prevention. In Chapter One the role of new mutations in maintaining the prevalence of genetic diseases in any human population was discussed, and it was noted that Down's syndrome prevalence is maintained largely by new mutations, with an inherited predisposition in a small percentage of cases. Down's syndrome would disappear if it were not constantly renewed by new mutations. Between 1 and 2 in 1,000 newborns suffer from Down's syndrome. About three-quarters of all cases of Down's syndrome conceived are lost by miscarriage. Down's syndrome is somewhat unusual in that a quarter are carried to term, as most chromosomal abnormalities of the embryo result in miscarriage with no survivors (Boué *et al.*, 1981a, 1981b).

The French Medical Research Council reported in 1970 that, using the characteristic markings of chromosomes, it was possible to say whether the extra chromosome in Down's syndrome had its origin at meiosis I or II (de Grouchy, 1970). Two years later two research workers at the Karolinska Hospital in Stockholm showed that the parental origin of the extra chromosome could be traced (Licznerski & Lindsten, 1972). In 1983 two paediatricians at the Children's Medical Center in Dayton, Ohio, summarized the results of 30 studies from Austria, Denmark, France, Netherlands and the U.S.A. Table 2.1 shows that of 369 cases of Down's syndrome 73.2 per cent originated at meiosis I and 26.8 per cent at meiosis II (Juberg & Mowrey, 1983). This is further evidence for the conclusion that Down's syndrome has its main origin in women during the 60 hours or so before ovulation. Juberg and Mowrey (1983) commented on the paternal responsibility for 20 per cent of cases:

'The fact that 20 per cent of the cases arose from spermatogenic nondisjunction has important implications. The first is that physicians and counsellors can help remove the onus that trisomy 21 syndrome is exclusively attributable to the mother. Second it should soon be possible to study a group of fathers for factors contributing to nondisjunction. Avoidance of an offending environmental agent might be possible after such studies.'

TABLE 2.1

ORIGINS OF DOWN'S SYNDROME IN GERM CELLS OF MOTHER OR FATHER; 369 CASES FROM 30 STUDIES, EUROPE AND U.S.A.

meiotic division	mother		father		both parents	
	N	%	N	%	N	%
first	225	61.0	45	12.2	270	73.2
second	67	18.1	32	8.7	99	26.8
total	292	79.1	77	20.9	369	100.0

Source: Juberg & Mowrey, 1983

The suggestion that nondisjunction may be caused by an 'offending environmental agent' is supported by reports that nondisjunction can be produced in animals by exposure to a variety of chemical compounds, about 20 having been listed by 1983 (Hansmann, 1984). A number of papers speculate as to whether nondisjunction is preceded by some genetic predisposition possibly caused by a mutation during the early production of the eggs in the female foetus. There is so far little evidence for such a predisposition, except in the 5 per cent or so of cases where the parent is carrying diagnosable chromosomal abnormalities. The animal experiments show moreover that nondisjunction can be produced at will by many different kinds of physical and chemical disturbance during the active stages of meiosis without predisposition, and nondisjunction is difficult to produce experimentally at any other time. Predisposition unless it can be diagnosed also offers little preventive opportunity and the safer hypothesis for a couple is that nondisjunction is caused not long before it happens during the highly susceptible periods around meiosis I and II. Chemicals that stop or slow down cell division, introducing a delay of a few hours, have been shown to increase the risk of nondisjunction in rat and Chinese hamster cells (Kamiguchi *et al.*, 1979). Chemicals that slow down cell division in this way include fungicides, organic solvents, anaesthetics, anti-cancer drugs and anti-anxiety drugs (Hsu *et al.*, 1983; Liang *et al.*, 1983). Diazepam (valium) was used by Hsu to stop cell division temporarily in female hamster cells. An arrest of cell division of 2 hours just before the final stages of meiosis I did not apparently damage the cells, but a temporary arrest of 7 hours resulted in many cells at subsequent divisions having the wrong number of chromosomes. In vivo temporary arrest of meiosis I and II may be caused by depression of the hypothalamic gonadal axis, for example by psychotropic drugs including alcohol (Gavaler & Van Thiel, 1987). The effects of such drugs are, however, distributed throughout the axis and it has been shown that alcohol can produce aneuploidy in mouse eggs after *in vivo* and *in vitro* activation with alcohol (Kaufman, 1985). Down's syndrome is discussed again in Chapter Eight in the context of ageing.

Apart from Down's syndrome the commonest diseases caused by chromosomal abnormalities are those involving the sex chromosomes, which are also mainly caused by one-generation inheritance from mother or father (Sperling, 1984). Both male and female sex chromosomal abnormalities have a frequency between 1.0 and 1.5 per 1,000 births (Buckton, 1983). The commonest abnormalities are Klinefelter's syndrome in boys and Turner's syndrome in girls, both associated with infertility. In all about 6 newborns in 1,000 have a recognizable chromosomal abnormality of which about 3 in 1,000 have some clinical significance. Six to ten per cent of stillborn infants and 5 to 7 per cent of children who die in infancy or early childhood have been reported to have chromosomal abnormalities (Hook, 1982).

SUSCEPTIBLE PERIOD IN WOMEN FOR THE ORIGIN OF MISCARRIAGE

An inherited propensity for any characteristic that increases infertility is unlikely to be common as it must tend to die out quickly. Among 24,951 American women undergoing amniocentesis it was found that about 5 in 1,000 were carrying translocations that might cause miscarriage (Hook *et al.*, 1984). A compilation of the cytogenetic findings of 79 published surveys of couples with two or more pregnancy losses showed an overall prevalence of chromosomal abnormalities of 2.8 per cent, a figure 5 or 6 times higher than the frequency in the general population of parents (Tharapel *et al.*, 1985). The results are summarised in Table 2.2 where it is seen that 31 per cent of the aberrations were carried by the men and 69 per cent by the women. Insofar as this 2.8 per cent of the couples owed their reduced fertility to inherited abnormal chromosomes the abnormalities must have been largely the result of new mutations in the germ cells of their own parents. In over 97.2 per cent of cases there was no evidence that the propensity was inherited by the couples who suffered the miscarriages.

Most miscarriages are a consequence of the fertilized ovum being defective. There have been a number of cytogenetic studies of aborted embryos. Carr

(1970) discussed the origin of many miscarriages in chromosomal abnormalities. Boué and Boué (1976) reported that 66 per cent of early spontaneous miscarriages before 8 weeks gestation had such chromosomal abnormalities. Poland *et al.* (1981) found 84 per cent of miscarried embryos less than 3mm long were abnormal and 57 per cent when karyotyped were found to be chromosomally abnormal. The data on some 5,000 miscarried embryos had been reported by 1981, and it is apparent from the chromosomal abnormalities alone that most of the defects in ova leading to miscarriage are already present in the zygotes immediately after fertilization and that they have their origin in male or female germ cells before fertilization. Most miscarriages of female origin begin during ovulatory maturation and an error at meiosis I, most frequently a nondisjunction, is the commonest cause of miscarriage.

TABLE 2.2

COUPLES WITH CHROMOSOMAL ABNORMALITIES FOUND AFTER TWO
OR MORE PREGNANCY LOSSES; 79 STUDIES

	women	men	total
number	8,208	7,834	16,042
number with abnormalities	319	143	362
per cent with abnormalities	3.9	1.8	2.8

Source: Tharapel *et al.*, 1985, Table 2, page 962.

Attempts have been made to prevent early miscarriage using hormones such as progesterone and drugs in early pregnancy. If in most cases of miscarriage the embryo is defective and the defects are already present in the zygote there is a danger that preventing miscarriage after fertilization will salvage defective embryos and increase the risk of a newborn with birth defects. Only intervention before conception, and, indeed, before ovulation can succeed in the primary prevention of miscarriage.

Hertig, an American pathologist at the Boston Lying-in Hospital, reported in the 1940s on 1,000 miscarriages and concluded that 62 per cent were connected with defects of the human ovum (Hertig & Sheldon, 1943). Twenty years later he published data indicating that these defects of the ovum had their origin before ovulation and were commoner if ovulation had been delayed (Hertig, 1967). He said in one of his papers that if in women the ovum lingers longer in the follicle than day 14 it has an increasing chance of becoming a 'defective ovum' when fertilized. The two lower rows in Figure 2.7 use Hertig's data and show the day of ovulation of normal and abnormal ova. The average time of ovulation of normal ova was 14 days and of abnormal ova 17 days. The upper row in Figure 2.7 shows the time of ovulation for pregnancies terminating in miscarriage (Iffy, 1981). The series of cases used to produce the upper row actually showed that premature ovulations as well as delayed ovulations were associated with miscarriages but the delayed ovula-

When ovulation is delayed

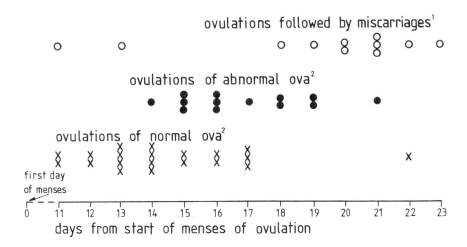

Figure 2.7. Miscarriage following delayed ovulation. Sources: Hertig, 1967, Table 2;
Iffy, 1981, Table 2; Wynn & Wynn, 1988a.

tions were commoner and appeared to be the greater risk. Evidence of the apparently damaging effect of delay in ovulation in women inspired animal experiments and several teams of investigators in different countries found that delay in ovulation increased the risk of chromosomal abnormalities (Bomsel-Helmreich *et al.*, 1979; Butcher & Fugo, 1967; Kamiguchi *et al.* 1979; Mikamo & Hamaguchi, 1975). New mutations were produced experimentally not by any direct poisoning of the ovum but by upsetting its hormone supplies during development. Butcher (1981) showed that a delay in ovulation for 48 hours in female rats caused a range of congenital malformations at every stage of embryonic and foetal development. Most of these malformations were not compatible with life but a small percentage were, and included abnormalities of the neural tube like spina bifida. The serious consequences of a delay of ovulation were similar whether or not the delay was caused by using drugs. If anything delays the LH surge meiosis and ovulation are delayed. It is seen in Figure 2.8 that in rat dams a low dose of smoke delayed the LH surge by about 1 hour and a high dose by about 2 hours (McLean *et al.*, 1977). The hypothalamus can delay or inhibit the LH surge. Nicotine in tobacco smoke is an example of many substances which act on the hypothalamus causing this delay. It is seen in Figure 2.9 that 3 doses of nicotine caused both a 2 hour delay in the LH surge and a depression to about half the normal level when injected into rat dams shortly before the normal time of the LH surge (Blake *et al.*, 1972). Four doses resulted in 5 hours' delay and a depression to only about a quarter of the normal level. High doses of a poison like nicotine

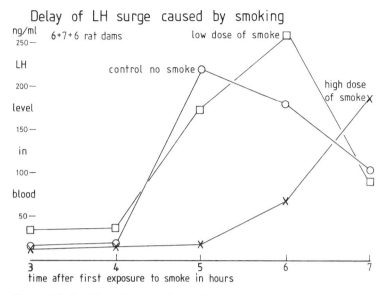

Figure 2.8. Smoking delays ovulation. Source: McLean et al., 1977, Figure 1. Reprinted by permission of Endocrinology, Williams and Wilkins.

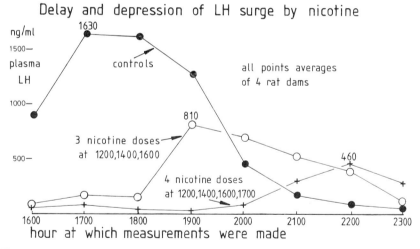

Figure 2.9. Nicotine depresses LH. Sources: Wynn & Wynn, 1988a, Figure 5. Blake *et al.*, 1972, Figure 1. Reprinted by permission of Endocrinology, Williams and Wilkins.

stop the LH surge altogether so that meiosis and ovulation stop and reproduction is prevented.

Drugs which affect the brain, including tranquillizers, narcotics, hypnotics, sedatives and alcohol, quite generally affect the secretion of sex hormones acting through the hypothalamus and pituitary glands (Smith, 1983). The exposure may not be severe enough to cause the hypothalamus to stop reproduction, but it may so affect follicular development as to prejudice the outcome after fertilization. Follicles, considering only size, can be either more or less grown. Follicles less than 16 mm in diameter at the time of ovulation are liable to die and disappear without producing a satisfactory, viable ovum. The normal range is 22 to 30 mm in diameter (Müller-Tyl *et al.*, 1984). The follicle has to reach a certain size for the ovum to survive. Less than satisfactory development of the follicle can prejudice subsequent development of the ovum (Bomsel-Helmreich *et al.*, 1979; Jongbloet, 1986). The granulosa cells produced during follicular development may be too few in number, too small or otherwise defective and produce an inadequate corpus luteum (Dizerega & Hodgen, 1981). After ovulation the granulosa cells stop dividing so the size of the corpus luteum is decided before ovulation. If the follicle is too small so is the corpus luteum.

Failure of the corpus luteum to provide an adequate supply of hormones, particularly progesterone but also oestrogens, is a mechanism of miscarriage following faulty follicular development because these hormones are essential to the first 6 to 7 weeks of pregnancy (Heap & Flint, 1984). If the hormones fail the pregnancy fails. During the first 8 weeks the placenta gradually takes over the task of supplying the hormones needed to maintain pregnancy and the corpus luteum is no longer needed from about the beginning of the third month of gestation. Anything that delays or depresses the supply of these pregnancy hormones is likely therefore to cause miscarriage. Smoking and exposure to nicotine would for this reason alone be expected to cause miscarriage as, indeed, it does, as shown in Figure 2.10 from a survey of smoking habits of women attending a New York hospital and their miscarriages compared to non-smokers.

The development of the embryo and placenta depends upon a blood supply containing adequate concentrations of hormones and nutrients including progesterone and oestrogens provided by the corpus luteum. An inadequate sup-

Smoking and the risk of miscarriage

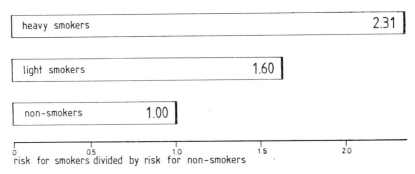

Figure 2.10. Smoking causes miscarriage. Source: Kline *et al.*, 1977, Table 1. Reprinted by permission of New England Journal of Medicine.

ply of hormones by the corpus luteum can slow down DNA synthesis and cell replication in the embryo. During the early stages of embryonic development the corpus luteum is also still dependent on luteotrophic hormones from the pituitary, so that anything that depresses the hypothalamic pituitary axis may also depress embryonic growth. However as the size of the corpus luteum is wholly determined during follicular development it is apparent that embryonic development has in some measure been already programmed before ovulation during growth of the follicle. As most chromosomal abnormalities have their origin at meiosis I before ovulation, and congenital malformations can be produced in animals by slowing down the growth of the follicle, the importance of normality of follicular development is apparent. The growth of the follicle is illustrated in Figure 2.11. The normal human follicle increases in diameter 12.5 times and in mass about 2,000 times in 14 days. This is the highest rate of growth found at any time during the human life cycle. Cell numbers in the follicle have to double about 11 times in 14 days, doubling once about every 30 hours. This is only possible if the follicle has a supply of blood with the right concentrations of hormones and nutrients and no poisons.

A high rate of follicular growth requires a high rate of synthesis of DNA. One cause of unsatisfactory pregnancy is a slow-down in rates of DNA synthesis beginning during ovulatory maturation in the female and extending through fertilization and embryonic development. The association of reduced mass of DNA in congenitally malformed pups and their placentas compared with normal pups is illustrated in Figures 2.12 & 2.13, based upon research by Potier de Courcy and colleagues at the French national laboratory for nutrition research (CNRS). The livers of the mothers of the malformed pups and their placentas had reduced DNA as shown in Figure 2.12. In this example the mothers were deprived of pantothenic acid and the foetal brain is seen to have been spared compared with the whole foetus or foetal liver, but neither foetus nor placenta were spared compared with the maternal liver (Potier de Courcy, 1966). Figure 2.13 shows the DNA content of malformed

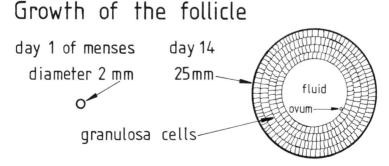

Figure 2.11. Source: Müller-Tyl *et al.*, 1984, Figure 10.
Reprinted by permission of Hemisphere Publishing Corporation.

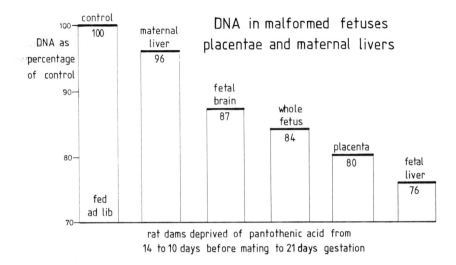

Figure 2.12. Association of malformation and reduced DNA caused by panthothenic deficiency. Source: Potier de Courcy, 1966, Tables 3 to 5.

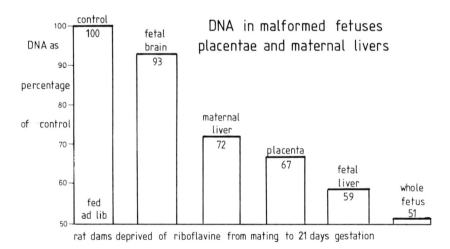

Figure 2.13. Association of malformation and reduced DNA caused by riboflavin deficiency. Sources: Potier de Courcy & Terroine, 1968, Tables 3 to 8; Potier de Courcy et al., 1970.

foetuses produced by riboflavin deficiency; the foetal brain is seen to have been spared compared with the maternal liver and indeed with the whole foetus and placenta (Potier de Courcy et al., 1970; Potier de Courcy et Terroine, 1968). In Figure 2.13 the deprivation only began at mating while in Figure 2.12 it began 14 to 10 days before mating. Different deficiencies with different time-scales are seen to produce different patterns of slow-down of DNA synthesis.

MOTHER, DAUGHTER, GRANDDAUGHTER

Susceptibility in the cycle of generations is shown diagrammatically in Figure 2.14. In the interests of simplicity this figure simplifies, some people may say oversimplifies, language. Twenty-four days after conception 'new ova' are shown in this figure to be visable. These new ova are the cells that carry the genetic code from one generation to the next, the germ cells. In a female embryo there are only around 100 of these new germ cells in the baby daughter's ova in Figure 2.14, 24 days after conception, but their number doubles about every 10 days to reach a maximum of about 7 million around the 6th month of gestation. Their number then begins to decline and continues to do so for the rest of the daughter's life so that few remain when she reaches 50. Of the 7 million new ova only one is needed for a mother eventually to have a granddaughter and a second to have a grandson and so for the next generation to be reproduced.

Cells are generally most susceptible to damage when dividing and it would therefore be expected that the immature ova in embryo or foetus would be most susceptible to damage during the first 6 months of the mother's pregnancy. Of these 6 months the first 2 are probably most susceptible. Attempts have been made to produce chromosomally abnormal young animals or embryos by exposing their germ cells early in their foetal existence to radiation but without success (Ivanov *et al.*, 1973). One study that also failed to produce any chromosomal abnormalities in offspring by irradiating their mothers early in pregnancy concluded that either the new ova at this stage were fairly resistant to radiation, or there was an efficient means of eliminating damaged

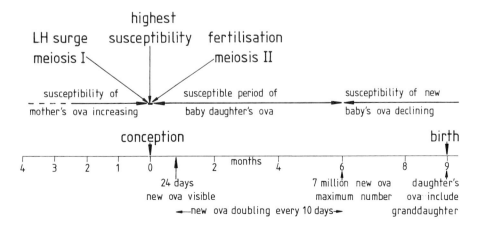

Figure 2.14. Female susceptibility through the generations.

cells, or there were effective repair mechanisms (Tsuchida & Uchida, 1974). These repair mechanisms and means of eliminating damaged cells are facilitated by the abundance of new ova produced. Commonsense suggests that ova may be damaged at any time from their first appearance. However, these ova lie dormant from 15 to 45 years in a mother's ovaries until their turn comes to ripen, and when dormant the chromosomes are tightly packed and apparently very resistant to any external influence.

However, both selection and repair mechanisms allow many kinds of abnormality to get through. The evidence that 2 or 3 per cent of miscarriages are at least partially caused by chromosomal abnormalities inherited from grandmothers shows that even such visible abnormalities sometimes get through, as do the gene defects inherited from grandparents and more remote forebears. Many mutations are copying errors that happen during cell division, and the high rates of cell division and DNA synthesis within the embryo during the first 8 weeks of pregnancy make this a time of enhanced risk not only to the next generation but also to the next but one.

3. Men's susceptibility before conception

CONGENITAL MALFORMATIONS CAUSED BY DAMAGE TO SPERM

Studies by Nomura at Osaka University summarised in Figures 2.5 and 2.6 showed that treatment of mouse sperm with radiation or chemicals can cause congenital malformations and cancer including leukaemia in offspring and some of the mutations are transmitted to the second generation (Nomura, 1975, 1978, 1982). Mary Lyon and her colleagues confirmed that irradiation of male or female mice before mating can lead to congenital malformations in offspring (Kirk & Lyon, 1982, 1984). The same team showed that, while some mutations can be passed on to the second generation by male offspring of irradiated parents, the major proportion of the malformations are eliminated in the first generation (Lyon & Renshaw, 1986, 1988). Adams *et al.* (1981) and Trasler *et al.* (1985) described foetal malformations and behavioural abnormalities following exposure of male mice before mating to cyclophosphamide. Nagao (1987) reported dose-dependent defects in offspring from treatment of male mice with MNU (methylnitrosourea). Russell and Hunsicker (1983) reported that exposure of sperm to MNU can produce specific locus mutations. Generoso *et al.* (1984) reported that exposure of sperm to MNU can produce heritable translocations. Mutation in male germ cells and the resulting abnormalities of offspring was the subject of a 144 page special issue of Mutation Research entitled 'Male-mediated F_1 abnormalities' (April 1990, Vol. 229, No 2). There is no evidence that male germ cells are any better protected than female germ cells from the ravages of mutagens.

It was suggested that the capacity of a substance to produce congenital defects in offspring by exposure of male sperm in animals should be used as a test of mutagenicity (Knudsen *et al.*, 1977). Not all the mutations produced in this way can be identified but those which can are generally found to be genetically dominant and autosomal. The consequences of such dominant mutations are diverse and difficult to identify. Testing has inevitably been generally restricted to the identification of dominant lethal mutations (Green *et al.*, 1985; Brusick, 1980; Burger *et al.*, 1989). Many hundreds of mutagens have been identified using the valuable dominant lethal test in which treated males are mated with untreated females and the resulting fertilised ova are examined for lethal defects. This test does not, however, identify many non-lethal dominant mutations such as those initiating viable malformations and tumour development. The first initiating mutation has been reported to be mainly of paternal origin in cases of inherited retinoblastoma and sporadic osteosarcoma (Ejima *et al.*, 1988; Schroeder *et al.*, 1987; Togucida *et al.*, 1989). A Medical Research Council team has suggested that leukaemia in children living near nuclear plants may be caused by their fathers' exposure to radiation resulting in germ cell mutations (Gardner *et al.*, 1990).

Abnormal sperm can cause miscarriage. Figure 3.1 shows an increasing risk of miscarriage with increasing sperm abnormality assessed using a phase contrast microscope: 200 cells were examined from specimens of semen from 317 men who were either husbands of women who had had miscarriages or were under investigation for infertility at hospitals in Stockholm (Furuhjelm *et al.*, 1962). Probably about half the miscarriages were attributable to the husband but the men in this study were in no sense representative. The same Swedish study showed that a low sperm concentration was also associated with an increased risk of miscarriage as illustrated in Figure 3.2. Low sperm concentration has been shown in other studies to be highly correlated with low percentages of morphologically normal sperm (Jouannet *et al.*, 1981). Volume of ejaculate is not reported to be associated with sperm quality so that sperm concentration may be more indicative than total sperm count. A slow-down in DNA synthesis and consequential reduction in the rate of cell replication could explain the copying errors associated with reduced rates of DNA synthesis. The increase in miscarriage rates is *prima facie* evidence that sperm abnormality may be associated with a raised mutation rate.

Research at the Ontario Cancer Institute showed that mutagens do indeed cause such sperm abnormalities visable under the microscope in animals (Wyrobek & Bruce, 1975). By 1982 tests had been done on 9 species of mammal including primates and 160 different chemicals (Wyrobek, 1982). The most

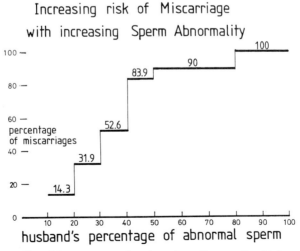

Figure 3.1. The quality of human semen in miscarriage. Source: Furuhjelm *et al.*, 1962, adapted from Figure 2.

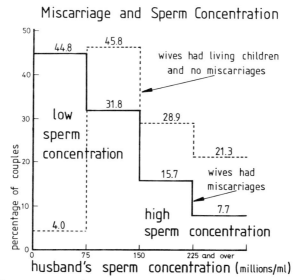

Figure 3.2. Sperm concentration and miscarriage. Source: Furuhjelm *et al.*, 1962, adapted from Figure 1.

sensitive visible indication of exposure to a mutagen is change in sperm shape. The head of the sperm is normally oval but may be too small, too large, round, double, narrow at the base, pear-shaped or the sperm may have an abnormal tail or two tails instead of one. In order to produce abnormalities of shape a mutagen must either damage the genes that determine shape or must affect the expression of these genes. Figure 3.3 shows the percentage of abnormal sperm produced by exposure to a mutagen at different times before ejaculation in rabbits (Fox *et al.*, 1963). It is seen that sperm shape is much more easily made abnormal by a mutagen before meiosis I and II. The sperm immediately after meiosis I and II is a spherical cell and sperm structure only develops subsequently at the spermatid stage. All the information necessary for pro-gramming sperm morphology is therefore carried by genes until the beginning of the spermatid stage. It is a reasonable inference that abnormal sperm mor-phology originating before meiosis I and II is a consequence of dominant gene mutations. This conclusion is supported by the long list of chemicals, known to be mutagens from other tests, that cause morphological sperm abnormality if fed to male animals. Morphological sperm abnormality has been shown not to be associated with chromosomal abnormality, further emphasizing that the morphological abnormality caused by mutagens must have its origin before the spermatid stage and before meiosis I and II as the result of dominant mutation of genes rather than chromosomal mutation (Martin & Rademaker, 1988).

In Figure 3.3 it is seen that the curve showing the percentage of abnormal sperm continues backwards in time until 70 days before ejaculation. In these

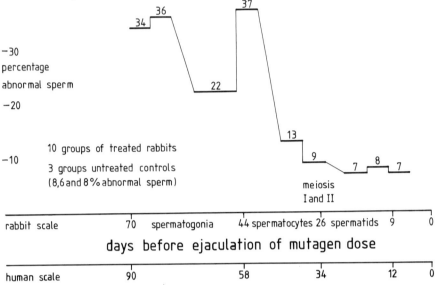

Figure 3.3. Source: Fox *et al.*, 1963, based on Table 2, column 1 for tretamine (0.2 mg/kg injected).

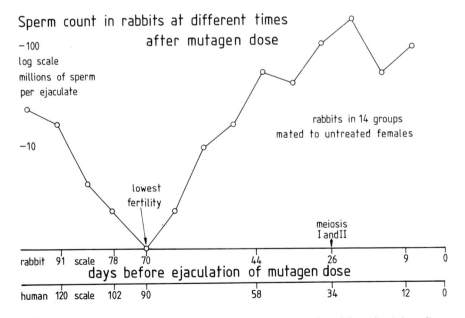

Figure 3.4. Fox *et al.*, 1963, based on Figure 1 for tretamine (0.2 mg/kg injected).

particular experiments with rabbits exposure to the mutagen 70 days before ejaculation stopped spermatogenesis. Figure 3.4 shows that 70 days before ejaculation was the point of maximum susceptibility, if measured in numbers of sperm per ejaculate. Comparing Figures 3.3 and 3.4 it is seen that the number of sperm declined as the percentage of abnormal sperm increased. At times longer that 70 days susceptibility to the mutagen dose declined and recovery from temporary infertility approached completion. The period of highest susceptibility in rabbits is seen to be well before meiosis I and II when the highest rates of DNA synthesis and cell replication take place. During this period germ cell numbers increase about 100 times. Spermatogonial replication ends when the germ cells are renamed spermatocytes about 35 days before ejaculation in mice, 44 days in rabbits and 58 days average in men as shown in Figure 3.5 in which the time-table of spermatogenesis is shown diagrammatically.

Spermatogenesis in all male mammals has a great power of recovery from temporary exposure to a mutagenic influence, but recovery takes time. In Figure 3.4 the 91 days for a rabbit and the 120 days for a man are indications of the minimum recovery times. There are many case histories showing times for recovery of sperm count following severe exposure to radiation or chemicals ranging up to 6 years, but there is generally no good information about the extent of the exposure. There may be no recovery of sperm count from very severe exposure (Whorton & Milby, 1980). Such severe exposure is, however, very uncommon. Temporary infertility resulting from interference with the replication of spermatogonia 2 or 3 months before attempts at conception are much commoner. The resistance of spermatogonial stem cells to mutagens continues to increase as the time interval to ejaculation increases beyond 120 days. This is apparent from case histories describing recovery after much longer intervals following exposure to radiation and chemicals. The existence of what have been called 'reserve stem cells' or 'spermatogonia A_0' that are isolated and rarely divide have been described in bulls, mice, monkeys and rats (Clermont & Bustos-Obregon, 1968; Clermont & Hermo, 1975). The existence of such resistant dormant male germ cells obviously had survival value like the resistant, dormant female germ cells more than a few months before ovulation.

THE TIME-TABLE OF SPERM SUSCEPTIBILITY

The longer the lapse of time between exposure to a mutagen and fertilization the greater is the opportunity for elimination or repair of a damaged germ cell. Figure 3.5 shows 58 ± 13 days from the end of spermatogonial cell replication until ejaculation. As less than 1 sperm in 10^9 ever fertilize an ovum the selection of less damaged sperm can offset effects of exposure to mutagens 2 or 3 months beforehand. The elimination of germ cells at every stage is

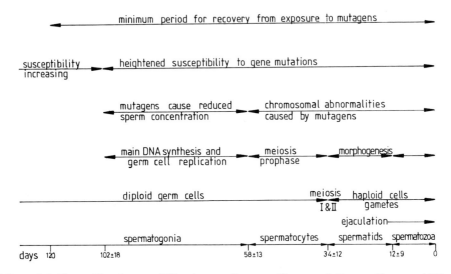

Figure 3.5. Time-table of susceptibility in men. Sources: Clermont & Bustos-Obregon, 1968; Heller & Clermont, 1964; Mann & Lutwak-Mann, 1981.

selective not random. Sperm with a very wide range of characteristics reducing viability fail to get through. Adler of the West German Institute of Genetics writes (Adler, 1983b):

> 'Chemically induced chromosomal changes in spermatogonia are eliminated by germinal selection. In contrast gene mutations are transmitted from stem-cell spermatogonia through meiosis to the offspring.'

This is illustrated in Figure 3.5. The dominant lethal test depends mainly on chromosomal changes. Such testing provides no information about the effect of mutagens on particular genes, which requires very large numbers of animals. An important study at the US Oak Ridge National Laboratory needed 304,479 mice offspring to study the mutation of only 7 genes (Russell, 1977). Such studies are costly and can never be done on men or women.

Gene mutations are thought to produce many more cases of congenital disorder than chromosomal mutations, but the evidence about causes is largely inferred from animal experiments and even then indirectly. It is inferred from animal experiments that mutagens can cause gene mutations that are responsible for morphological abnormality of sperm. Because gene mutations may have an immense variety of consequences which are impossible to identify in routine testing there is a danger that the length of the period of heightened susceptibility may be underestimated. The chromosomal abnormalities produced by the drug mitomycin C in mice is illustrated in Figure 3.6. It is seen that no chromosomal abnormalities were recorded in the mice as resulting from a mutagen dose more than 27 days before mating (Ehling, 1971). This limitation to 27 days is seen in Figure 3.7 to be the result of failure to survive of any sperm produced more than 31 days before mating. Figure 3.8 shows another susceptibility-time curve based on studies at the US Oakridge National Laboratory using a chemical (MMS) that affects primarily the spermatid stage (Brewen *et al.*, 1975). Such susceptibility time-curves are only available for a few drugs and chemicals, are unpredictable and expensive to produce. The practical conclusion is that when such information is not available any drug or chemical should be assumed to be able to produce chromosomal abnormalities in offspring from early in the spermatocyte stage but not longer, that is up to 58±13 days before ejaculation in men or not longer than 12 weeks.

Ehling and Neuhäuser-Klaus (1988) of the West German Institute for Mammalian Genetics compared the data for cyclophosphamide for dominant lethal mutations and specific-locus gene mutations in experiments involving an examination of a total of 248,413 mouse pups. The susceptibility-time curves for dominant-lethal mutations were not very different from Figure 3.8 for MMS. Moreover susceptibility to gene mutations at 7 specific loci was highest during the 21 days before mating and after meiosis. When, however, the effect of cyclophosphamide was enhanced with X-rays the period of heightened susceptibility increased to about 42 days before mating to include spermatocytes and differentiating spermatogonia, and there were a few mutations at even longer intervals. The period of enhanced susceptibility to gene mutations may be at least twice as long as for dominant lethal mutations and chromosomal abnormalities as suggested in Figure 3.5. and begins well before the first cell divisions of spermatogenesis.

The experiments of Nomura (1982) described in Chapter Two and illustrated in Figure 2.5 and 2.6 showed no significant increase in dominant lethal mutations following exposure of spermatogonia to either radiation or urethane. But such exposure resulted in an increase in malformations and tumours in surviving pups not caused, in Nomura's words, by 'gross chromosomal changes' but by dominant gene mutations. Nomura pointed to greater susceptibility of the postmeiotic stages, but also said that the spermatocytes were most susceptible to radiation '22 to 42 days before mating' without however giving the data.

The time-table of human sperm development summarized in Figure 3.5 shows the length of the period of heightened susceptibility to gene mutations as 102 days. This is a conservative figure based on the studies of Heller and Clermont (1964) in the U.S.A. and Canada. They estimated the duration of sperm development at 90 days, to which a variable period of storage of the finished spermatozoa has to be added. An average period of 12 days has been estimated (Harper, 1982). The length of storage falls as sexual activity increases and may be as short as 3 days (Mann & Lutwak-Mann, 1981). The

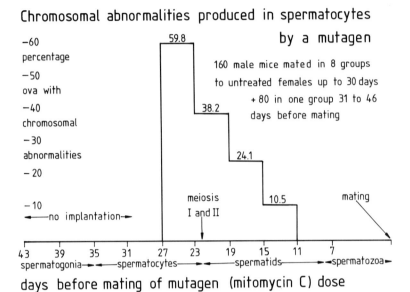

Figure 3.6. Dominant lethal mutations produced around meiosis I and II.
Source: Ehling, 1971, Table IV.

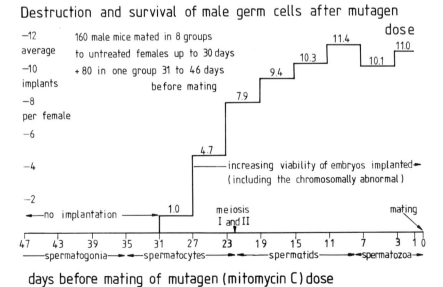

Figure 3.7. Destruction of spermatogonia by mutagen. Source: Ehling, 1971, Table IV.

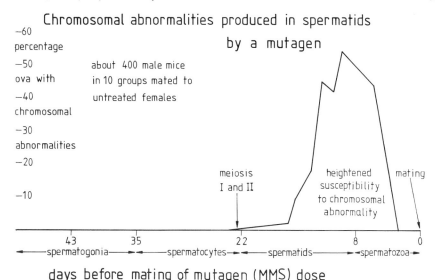

Figure 3.8. Dominant lethal mutations produced by post-meiotic exposure of male germ cells. Source: Brewen *et al.*, 1975, Table 1.

viability of the spermatozoa within the epididymis probably lasts for at least 3 weeks. The storage period of the spermatozoa may therefore be said to be 12 days with a tolerance of ±9 days.

The number of male germ cells, and the amount of new DNA, reach a maximum at the beginning of the spermatocyte stage, 58±13 days before ejaculation when all replication stops. The tolerances shown in Figure 3.5 mainly reflect the variable storage time in the epididymis. The peak of susceptibility for gene mutations may be around 80 to 90 days before ejaculation. The decline in susceptibility to mutagens going backwards in time to 120 days before ejaculation is substantial. Four months is a conservative estimate of the time needed for male reproductive capacity to recover from a not very potent dose of mutagen. Because the susceptible periods for mutagens vary widely, and are generally unpredictable, longer rather than shorter periods have been chosen when in doubt so that Figure 3.5 should cover most causes of mutation. Russell, who was quoted in Chapter Two as emphasizing the importance of the great increase in susceptibility in the female during ovulatory maturation, has also emphasized the susceptibility of the male to chemical mutagens during spermatogenesis (Russell, 1986). Mary Lyon said when discussing chemical mutagens (Lyon, 1988):

'The major part of the data available concerns males, and the majority of the chemicals tested so far fall in the category of those that have little effect on the spermatogonial stem cells. Thus, for these it is only any dose received in a few weeks or months before conception that need be considered.'

Spermatogonial stem cells may be damaged by radiation and by some chemicals but a high proportion of all mutations in men happen later, during the susceptible periods before conception.

HEIGHTENED SUSCEPTIBILITY IMMEDIATELY BEFORE CONCEPTION

The effects of exposure to mutagens immediately before mating have been studied. The mutagenic effect of a drug, fosfestrol, on male mice, as indicated by the fertilized ova found to be lethally damaged, is shown in Figure 3.9 from Ehling (1979). Batches of 40 male mice were mated at different time intervals between dosing and mating to healthy undosed females. Drugs given to male animals immediately before mating can cause congenital malformations, reduced birthweight, small litters, stillbirths and reduced neonatal survival. This effect is not necessarily a result of the reaction of the drug with the male germ cell, as it has been shown by Lutwak-Mann (1964) in research at Cambridge that drugs can be carried by sperm into the female tract to the point of fertilization where they can cause congenital malformations. Exposure of sperm to thalidomide has been shown to cause congenital malformations in this way (Lutwak-Mann, 1964; Lutwak-Mann *et al.*, 1967).

The interest in these experiments is not in the drug but in the effects on offspring of drugging sperm. The effects of methadone on sperm have been studied at the University of Vermont (Soyka & Joffe, 1980). Methadone given to male rats during the 24 hours before mating caused an increase in the percentage of pups born dead from 13 to 54 per cent as shown in Figure 3.10. The pups born alive following drugging of the male sperm also had reduced viability as shown in Figure 3.11 which also shows that morphine had a similar effect. It is seen in Figure 3.11 that nearly 100 per cent of control pups survived, but only 65 per cent of pups from males dosed with morphine, and 28

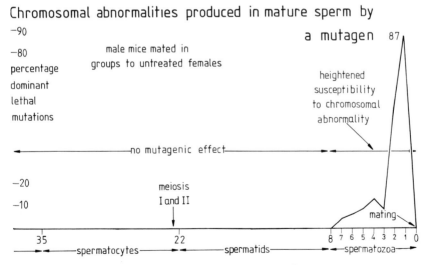

Figure 3.9. Dominant lethal mutations produced by exposure of spermatozoa.
Sources: Ehling, 1979, Table 1; Wynn & Wynn, 1989.

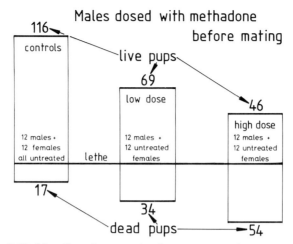

Males dosed with methadone before mating

live pups

Figure 3.10. Mortality of rat pups by drug treatment of male before mating.
Source: Soyka & Joffe, 1980, Figure 2.

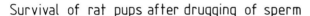

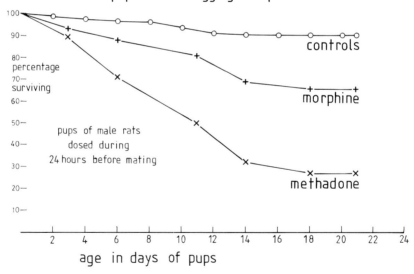

Survival of rat pups after drugging of sperm

Figure 3.11. Viability of rat pups reduced by drug treatment of male before mating.
Sources: Soyka & Joffe, 1980, Figure 1; Wynn & Wynn, 1989.

per cent of pups from males dosed with methadone survived the first 20 days of life. Both stillbirths and neonatal deaths followed the drugging of sperm. These drugs must either have damaged the male genetic code shortly before fertilization or must have caused genetic damage around the time of fertilization or shortly afterwards. Both methadone and morphine have been shown in other studies to be mutagenic and Figures 3.10 and 3.11 may be regarded as further evidence of their mutagenicity (Badr & Rabouh, 1983; Badr *et al.*, 1979). The common analgesic codeine, found in many non-prescription pain-killers, is a derivative of morphine and morphine is one of the metabolic products of codeine which must therefore also be assumed to be mutagenic. Codeine has been reported in other experiments to cause congenital malformations (Zellers & Gautieri, 1977).

THE COMPARATIVE SUSCEPTIBILITY OF MEN AND WOMEN

It has been suggested by a number of writers that new mutations in surviving children may be more frequently of male than female origin, because the male germ cell undergoes many more cell divisions than the female germ cell and most new mutations are thought to be the result of copying errors during division (Vogel, 1984). The larger number of male germ cells facilitates more effective germinal selection which eliminates chromosomal abnormalities produced during the replication of the spermatogonia at the beginning of spermatogenesis. Germinal selection is not, however, so effective in eliminating dominant gene mutations. 1,443 (+ 1,114 not fully validated) dominant genetic disorders which are distinctive have so far been listed and the commoner disorders which reduce fertility have their population prevalence maintained by new mutations (McKusick, 1988). Dominant autosomal mutations are discussed again in Chapter Eight in the context of ageing.

There is a longer period in the man of 34 ± 12 days from meiosis I and II to fertilization than in a woman which may explain, for example, the 80 per cent maternal and 20 per cent paternal origin of Down's syndrome. However in a study of triploidy, a major cause of miscarriage, 72 per cent of cases were reported to be of paternal origin (Sperling, 1984). In Klinefelter's syndrome, which seriously affects male sexual development, there is an extra X chromosome which was reported to have its origin at meiosis I in the father in about one third of a series of cases (Sanger *et al.*, 1977). A study from the University of Oregon (1980) of 42 other chromosomal rearrangements found that 22 were of maternal and 19 of paternal origin (Chamberlin & Magenis, 1980; Mattei *et al.*, 1982); the chromosomal abnormalities originating in the father were mostly a consequence of chromosomal breakage and rejoining at the wrong place.

It is currently a cautious and wise assumption that men and women have germ cells equally vulnerable. This is the conclusion of several studies that have emphasized the difficulty of any comparison of the responsibilities of mothers and fathers for an unfavourable pregnancy outcome caused by damage to germ cells (Adler, 1982a, 1982b, 1982c). The male time-table of susceptibility differs from that of the female and is more complicated and varies from one mutagen to the next making comparisons difficult. Some one-generation genetic disease is more paternal and some more maternal in origin. The International Commission of the Mutagen Societies (1983) discussing short-term exposure of men and women concluded that:

'It may be particularly important to know the risk to maturing germ cells (in men and women), since it may be possible to avoid the genetic harm done to these stages if the accidentally exposed individuals refrain from conception for 3 months'.

Where possible exposure to X-rays or drugs should be avoided during the 3 or 4 months before conception. Risk is, however, a product of susceptibility, enhanced during this period of the maturing cell, and the exposure to mutagenic influences of all kinds. The literature assumes that everyone has a general mutation rate affecting both somatic and germ cells. The concept of a mutation rate is not without difficulties but is useful. The reproductive risk is then the product of this mutation rate and an enhancement factor depending upon time of exposure. The reproductive risk is obviously zero for someone beyond reproductive age, but greatly enhanced for men and women around the time of conception.

Chapters Two and Three have discussed this enhancement of susceptibility and have only discussed factors that increase mutation such as X-rays or drugs in order to illustrate this enhancement more particularly during the period immediately before conception. The rest of this book is primarily concerned with the ever increasing number of factors that are known both to increase and also to reduce human mutation rates.

4. Effects of nutrient imbalance on reproduction

MUTATIONS CAUSED BY FOLIC ACID DEFICIENCY

Pernicious anaemia appears to have been the first well-known human disorder shown to be associated with the production of chromosomal abnormalities and an increased human mutation rate. The knowledge that anaemia and other illness was associated with visible damage to the cell nucleus goes back to the 19th century. Fragments of the cell nucleus found within red blood cells were discussed in 1899 by Schmauch of the Royal Pathological Institute of Königsberg. His 20-item bibliography from 1865 includes many descriptions of the occurrence of these fragments in animals and humans associated with illness. Following a paper by Howell (1890), an American physiologist, these nuclear fragments became known as 'Howell's bodies', or sometimes as Howell-Jolly bodies. Jolly (1905) being a French histologist who also described these microscopic particles. Although the appearance and even the number of these particles depends upon the techniques used for their study they are essentially the same particles described today as micronuclei.

More than half a century later Hutchison and Ferguson-Smith (1959) from the University of Glasgow published a paper on the significance of Howell-Jolly bodies which they had identified in 52 consecutive cases of pernicious anaemia. It was well-known by 1959 that pernicious anaemia could be produced by deficiencies of folic acid or of cobalamin (B_{12}). Chromosomes were first described in 1873 and acquired their name in 1888 and their functions were broadly understood by the turn of the century. Hutchison and Ferguson-Smith appear, however, to have been the first to draw the separate lines of investigation together and to conclude that Howell-Jolly bodies were partly composed of chromosome fragments and were formed as a result of nutrient deficiencies. Hutchinson & Ferguson-Smith concluded:

> 'It seems probable that disordered nucleic acid synthesis resulting from B_{12} or folic acid deficiency is the fundamental factor in the production of this abnormal behaviour at mitosis.'

Potier de Courcy (1966) of the University of Paris showed that in rats folic acid deficiency slows down synthesis in the embryo of DNA, RNA and protein. Papers from a number of countries showed that there was an association between folic acid or cobalamin deficiency and chromosomal damage in somatic cells, generally blood cells (Astaldi *et al.*, 1962; Forteza & Baguena,

1963; Kiossoglou *et al.*, 1965; Heath, 1966; Menzies *et al.*, 1966; Bottura & Coutinho, 1967). It was confirmed by these investigators that Howell-Jolly bodies or micronuclei could be produced by nutrient deficiencies, and that a range of chromosomal abnormalities could be produced by folic acid or co-balamin deficiency which were mutagenic at least in somatic cells. Heath (1966) reported that cobalamin and folic acid deficiency in cell culture in-creased chromosome breakage but without producing any characteristic, rec-ognizable type of aberration. Menzies *et al.* (1966) found that cobalamin and folic acid deficiency caused 'numerous morphological abnormalities' of chro-mosomes. Hall and Davidson (1968) referred to the 'widespread cytological dystrophy' caused by folic acid deficiency. A later paper noted that a folic acid antagonist could cause breakage of any chromosome and could cause single or multiple breaks or 'total fragmentation or pulverization' (Mandello *et al.*, 1984). Folic acid deficiency has been shown to cause nondisjunction in mice (Gates *et al.*, 1981).

Stevenson (1978) described the effects of 12 folic acid analogues which behave like folic acid antagonists producing the symptoms of folic acid defi-ciency. Methotrexate and aminopterin are perhaps the best known of these folic acid antagonists. Stevenson showed, as would be expected, that 11 out of 12 of these compounds produced chromosomal abnormalities in human lymphocytes in cell culture. All effects of these compounds could be prevented with tetrahydrofolic acid, the active reduction product of folic acid and also by thymine, one of the essential DNA bases requiring folic acid for its syn-thesis. The frequency of occurrence of micronuclei, or Howell-Jolly bodies, in the cells from normal individuals cultured in a medium deficient in folic acid or thymidine or both is shown in Figure 4.1. (Jacky *et al.* 1983). The number of micronuclei is seen to have been 10 times higher in the medium deficient in both these nutrients which appear to be interchangeable in this

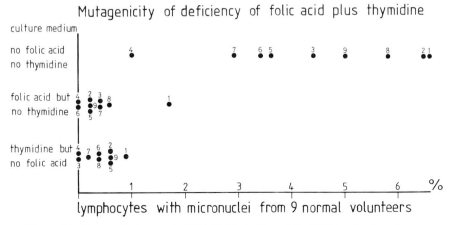

Figure 4.1. Source: Jacky *et al.*, 1983, Table 1. Copyright 1983 by the American Association for the Advancement of Science.

special context. Similar studies have been published by Reidy *et al.* (1983) of the US Center for Environmental Health, Georgia. The frequency of occurrence of chromosomal breaks in the cultured cells of 25 normal individuals is shown in Figure 4.2 and of chromosomal gaps in Figure 4.3. In both cases the frequency of chromosomal abnormalities is compared for cells cultured in media containing and not containing folic acid. The authors comment that the variations between people in their chromosomal breakage rates may be caused by their different folic acid status, but also by other differences in the composition of their blood plasma or intracellular fluids.

It is apparent that folic acid deficiency increases mutation rates which would be expected to cause infertility when it seriously affects germ cells. Mathur *et al.* (1977), reported on the effects of folic acid deficiency produced by aminopterin, one of the folic acid antagonists, on spermatogenesis in male albino rats. Aminopterin was used in doses too low to produce any overt toxic effects. Spermatogenesis was affected within 7 days and changes in blood cells and bone marrow in 15 days. The authors commented:

'This finding indicates that the testis is even more sensitive to folic acid deficiency than is hemopoietic tissue.'

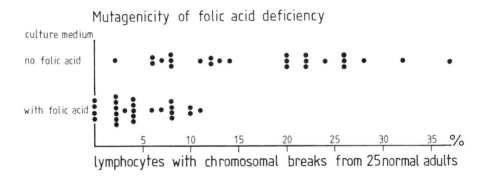

Figure 4.2. Source: Reidy *et al.*, 1983, Table 1.

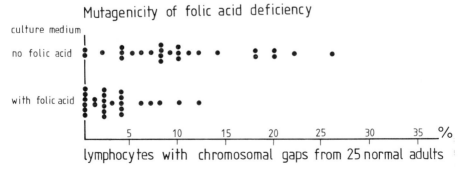

Figure 4.3. Source: Reidy *et al.*, 1983, Table 1.

The folic acid deficiency resulted in the production of chromosomal abnormalities and a progressive reduction in the number of sperm cells at all stages of development as the deficiency continued. Folic acid antagonists used medicinally have been reported to cause large reductions in sperm counts in male patients (Sussman & Leonard, 1980).

Adams (1958) had reported in the Scottish Medical Journal that involuntary infertility was a 'striking feature' common to a series of women patients with pernicious anaemia. A number of studies followed of infertility in men associated with cobalamin deficiency. Watson (1962) reported the association of low seminal cobalamin with sterility and morphological abnormalities of sperm. This association of sperm quality and motility with cobalamin concentration had at this time already been reported in the veterinary literature, for example, as influencing the fertility of bulls (Busch, 1954). Sharp and Witts (1962) of the Radcliffe Infirmary, Oxford, pointed out that damage to sperm in men predated symptoms of anaemia suggesting that germ cells are more sensitive to deficiency of cobalamin than the cells of the bone marrow:

'It is well known that pernicious anaemia may be present in a latent form for some years before giving rise to symptoms of anaemia. The vitamin B_{12} in the serum should therefore always be estimated when unexplained impairment of spermatogenesis is found.'

Adams (1958) had reported that sterility associated with subclinical anaemia in women preceded overt symptoms by a long period and this was confirmed by Smith (1962) who concluded:

'It seems desirable to screen all patients, both male and female, with unexplained sterility for subclinical evidence of Addisonian anaemia.'

Such screening depends upon definitions and acceptance of 'subclinical evidence' of a damaging deficiency. Megaloblastic anaemia has been regarded as the definitive evidence of cobalamin and folic acid deficiencies. However, deficiencies of these nutrients have been reported to be associated with pathological consequences without being sufficiently severe to produce megaloblastic changes in blood cells. Thus Tomaszewsky *et al.* (1963) published data showing that semen cobalamin concentrations associated with oligospermia and azospermia were below average but were not as low as would be expected for patients with overt megaloblastic anaemia. The greater sensitivity of germ cells compared with bone-marrow cells to moderate deficiencies of cobalamin could explain the sterility that precedes megaloblastic anaemia by months or even years. Other body systems including the immune system and central nervous system are affected by marginal deficiencies of both cobalamin and folic acid insufficient to produce anaemia.

Steinberg *et al.* (1983), of the Universities of Minnesota and Washington used radioactive labelled folic acid cells cultured in the laboratory. A critical level of intracellular folic acid concentration was found of $0.1 ng/10^6$ cells below which DNA replication and cell division cease. Only below this level do 'bizarre multinucleate cells' and megaloblastosis become apparent. However intracellular concentrations above this threshold in the range 0.1 to $0.5ng/10^6$ cells are associated with abnormalities of DNA synthesis. Megaloblastic anaemia is seen to be evidence only of extreme folic acid deficiency, and there are less serious levels of deficiency that still interfere with DNA synthesis. The morphological criteria of deficiency are much less sensitive than biochemical criteria. In more usual units, not used by Steinberg, there is a risk of megaloblastic anaemia at intracellular concentrations below about 140ng/ml, but of some interference with DNA synthesis up to much higher concentrations diminishing with increase in concentrations up to 3 or 4 times this figure. The 140ng/ml is the usually accepted 'high risk' threshold (Sauberlich *et al.*, 1977).

NUTRITIONAL DEFICIENCY DURING PERIODS OF HIGH SUSCEPTIBILITY

In the 1940s and 1950s there were three important research centres studying the effects of nutritional deficiencies on reproduction, in France at the Medical School of the University of Paris, in Switzerland at the University of Geneva and in the USA at the University of California. All these centres showed that in female animals deficiencies of essential nutrients could affect fertility and the health of offspring. Watteville *et al.* (1954) of the University of Geneva showed that a deficiency of any one of the four B vitamins thiamin, riboflavin, pyridoxine or pantothenic acid beginning 13 days before mating reduced the fertility of rat dams by up to 80 per cent and beginning 28 days before mating by 100 per cent. By 1951 it had already been shown that a deficiency of vitamin A could cause both infertility and congenital malformations (Hale, 1933). It had also been shown that a deficiency of folic acid could cause infertility and malformations (Nelson & Evans, 1949; Giroud & Lefebvres-Boisselot, 1951). Ross and Pike (1956) of Pennsylvania State University showed that rats deprived of pyridoxine before mating produced pups of low birthweight even when pyridoxine was restored to the diet immediately after mating. They concluded:

> 'The data indicate that pyridoxine in the diet before mating is as important as pyridoxine in the diet during gestation; giving further support to the hypothesis that the condition of the maternal organism prior to the inception of pregnancy plays a critical role in the course of pregnancy and its outcome.'

Nelson and Evans (1955) of the University of California found that thiamin deficiency initiated 11 to 15 days before mating caused 83 per cent of embryos to be resorbed as illustrated in Figure 4.4. If the deficiency was initiated earlier still most animals had no implantations. Thiamin deprivation before mating resulted in low birthweight among surviving pups of the deficient dams as illustrated in Figure 4.5. It was not very clear in any of these experiments just

Thiamin deficiency before mating and infertility

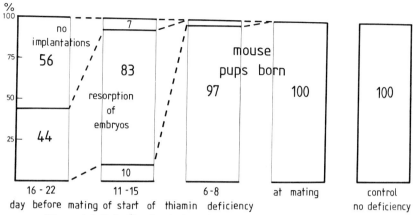

Figure 4.4. Infertility by timing of thiamin deficiency in rat dams.
Source: Nelson & Evans, 1955, Table 1.

Thiamin deficiency before mating and birthweight

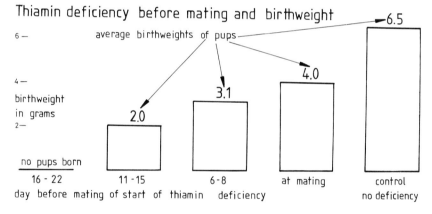

Figure 4.5. Low birthweight by timing of maternal thiamin deficiency in rats.
Source: Nelson & Evans, 1955, Table 1.

when the induced deficiencies had their physiological effects, but the effects were most marked when the nutritional deficiency began before mating and if begun early enough it always inhibited ovulation. If the deficiencies were initiated somewhat later nearer mating ovulation proceeded but implantation was inhibited, or if implantation proceeded the embryo could be malformed or be resorbed.

The deficiency needed to produce these results was modest. Riboflavin deficiency was reported to cause malformations in rats by Warkany and Schraffenberger in 1943. The same authors said in a later paper (Warkany & Schraffenberg, 1944):

'We are dealing in these experiments with a borderline deficiency … Abnormal offspring appear when the riboflavin of the blood reaches a certain critical level. A reduction of

riboflavin below the critical level leads to sterility and embryonic death, while an increase
beyond this level results in the birth of normal young.'

Warkany was a pioneer in the study of causes of congenital malformations
(Warkany, 1971). Giroud *et al.* (1949, 1950, 1952) pursued research on riboflavin deficiency at the Medical School of the University of Paris. Giroud
failed to produce any malformations by depriving female rats of riboflavin
beginning only from or after mating, but a high percentage of resorbed embryos and malformed young were produced when riboflavin deprivation began
11 to 22 days before mating as shown in Figure 4.6. Giroud measured the
extent of the maternal riboflavin depletion associated with various pregnancy
outcomes which are summarized in Table 4.1. It is seen in Table 4.1 that
riboflavin deficiency caused low birthweight, malformation or resorption of
offspring at levels which caused no maternal signs.

Riboflavin and pantothenic acid are both coenzymes and animal reproduction has been reported to be upset if enzyme saturation falls below about 80
per cent (Esch *et al.*, 1981). Levels of enzyme saturation appear to correspond
approximately to the percentage liver contents in Table 4.1 and are in practice
easier to measure. Eighty per cent instead of 100 per cent enzyme saturation
would not be expected to produce signs of deficiency as tissues generally have
enzyme reserves. Some explanation is needed of the susceptibility of the reproductive system to such a modest depression of enzyme saturation levels
and to nutrient deficiencies that would not be noticed outside reproduction.
The explanation is to be found in the susceptibility of the endocrine system
to nutrient deficiencies discussed further below.

Later research by Potier de Courcy and Terroine (1968) also of the Paris
Medical School confirmed Giroud's findings and referred to six other studies

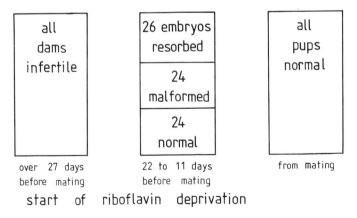

Figure 4.6. Malformations and infertility by timing of riboflavin deficiency in rat dams.
Source: Giroud *et al.*, 1952, Table 2.

TABLE 4.1

RIBOFLAVIN DEPLETION IN MATERNAL RAT LIVER FOR DIFFERENT
PREGNANCY OUTCOMES: ALL ANALYSES AT 21 DAYS' GESTATION

	maternal liver riboflavin as percentage of normal 45 mcg/g
normally fed controls	100
outcome when deprived 4 or more days before mating:	
low birthweight pups	80
congenitally malformed pups	65
abortion or resorption	54
maternal signs of riboflavin deficiency	50
maternal death	35

Source: Giroud *et al.*, 1949.

describing the modesty (légèreté) of the deficiency needed to cause malformations. Pantothenic acid deficiency was also shown to produce malformed foetuses in 100 days without there being any 'external signs' of deficiency. These experiments showed that rats and mice were more susceptible to damage from nutrient deficiency before and around the time of mating than at any other time in the life cycle. The same deficiencies later in pregnancy, or in young or adults, produced no apparent effects.

Giroud *et al.*, (1950) also noted that the mother early in pregnancy had priority for riboflavin over the foetus. During the latter part of pregnancy, including human pregnancy, the placenta extracts vitamins from the maternal serum for the benefit of the foetus. The human baby has a higher blood serum riboflavin than his mother (van den Berg *et al.*, 1978). The placental pump, so important in all the later stages of pregnancy, does not exist in the early stages which are therefore less protected. This was not understood by the early investigators, nor was it at first understood how the endocrine system enhances susceptibility to some nutrient deficiencies.

HORMONAL IMBALANCE CAUSED BY NUTRITIONAL DEFICIENCIES

Nelson *et al.* (1951, 1953) found that by injection of the ovarian hormones oestrone and progesterone they could restore the fertility of rat dams made infertile by pyridoxine deficiency before mating. They also found that injection of gonadotrophins (LH, FSH, prolactin) restored implantations to 78 per cent of controls but only 29 per cent had living young. Nelson (1953) concluded:

'Dysfunction of both the pituitary and the ovary is involved in the hormonal inadequacies of these vitamin-deficient animals.'

Nelson and Evans (1955) found the effects of thiamin deficiency before mating illustrated in Figures 4.4 and 4.5 could be prevented and fertility could be restored by injection daily of 1mcg oestrone and 4mg of progesterone.

It was concluded from these studies that the endocrine system mediates the effects of many nutrient deficiencies and inhibits reproduction before these deficiencies have any direct effect on germ cells or embryo. All nutrient deficiencies do not however act in this way. Thus the effects of folic acid or pantothenic acid deficiency on reproduction cannot be corrected by injection of hormones (Nelson *et al.*, 1951). The secretion of many hormones is modulated by nutrition including for example growth hormone, somatomedins and insulin (Phillips & Vassilopoulou-Sellin, 1979). However the level of gonadotrophins appears to be affected at lesser degrees of nutrient deficiency than other hormones. In the course of evolution this characteristic probably had survival value preventing reproduction when food supplies were unsatisfactory. In the context of reproduction the endocrine system became the arbiter of nutritional adequacy. Ovulation ceased or implantation failed long before there was any real threat to the female. Luteinizing hormone (LH) appears to be depressed by an inadequate diet.

The effects of different nutrient deficiencies on hormonal balance need further study and are complicated by feed-back for example between ovarian hormones and the hypothalamus, which is part of the normal control of hormone levels. Riboflavin deficiency causes hormonal imbalance illustrated for oestradiol and progesterone in Figures 4.7 and 4.8 based on experiments on gilts by Esch *et al.* (1981) of the University of Illinois. Riboflavin is essential

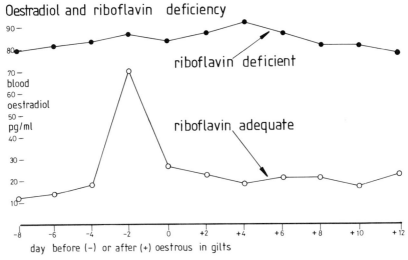

Figure 4.7. Disturbance of oestradiol levels in pigs. Source: Esch *et al.*, 1981, Figure 2.

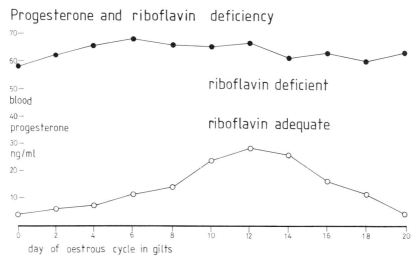

Figure 4.8. Disturbance of progesterone levels in pigs. Source: Esch *et al.*, 1981, Figure 3.

for the homeostasis and liver clearance of these steroid hormones and a deficiency causes excessive accumulation which inhibits LHRH secretion by the hypothalamus and gonadotrophin secretion by the pituitary with resulting infertility.

As discussed further below low maternal energy intake or protein intake also cause hormonal imbalance. During the early stages of reproduction including both ovulatory maturation and spermatogenesis a normal hormonal profile is a primary requirement of satisfactory reproduction. A defective diet is a diet that causes hormonal imbalance.

HORMONAL IMBALANCE CAN BE MUTAGENIC

In a symposium entitled 'Mutations in Man' (Obe, 1984) Hansmann of the University of Göttingen suggested that failures of neuroendocrine control are a primary cause of chromosomal abnormalities and in particular of nondisjunction at meiosis I which happens in females during follicular development and concluded:

'Such alterations in normal follicular function may result from various failures at any level of the hypothalamic-pituitary-gonadal axis.'

In particular reduced levels of gonadotrophins slow down follicular development, delay ovulation, and thereby increase the risk of error at meiosis I.

Individual hormones have been shown to be mutagenic in excess and also when deficient. Oestradiol, although an essential ovarian hormone, has been shown to be mutagenic in excess in mice and in human lymphocyte culture

(Banduhn & Obe, 1985; Becker & Schönreich, 1981). Progesterone in excess has been shown to be mutagenic in male and female animals including dogs, hamsters and rats. Excess progesterone interferes with meiosis in male and female animals and can cause a variety of trisomies and monosomies. The general effect of excess progesterone is to make animals infertile, but the animal experiments show that some cells with chromosomal abnormalities remain viable and proceed through meiosis although defective (Williams *et al.*, 1971).

Lucille Hurley, of the University of California and one-time President of the Teratology Society, suggested that any factor that reduces embryonic DNA synthesis increases the risk of malformations (Eckhert & Hurley, 1977; Hurley, 1981). Most congenital malformations are associated with total numbers of cells and not reduced cell size. A slow-down in rates of cell replication caused by a slow-down in DNA synthesis increases the risk of disorganized differential growth and malformations. When the slow-down can be prevented by injection of ovarian hormones it is reasonable to conclude that it is a shortage of these hormones that is responsible for the slow-down, the growth disorganization and malformations. During early embryonic development immediately following fertilization progesterone is the hormone likely to be in short supply and to have these effects. Progesterone deficiency is a consequence of the corpus luteum having too few cells because of too low a rate of replication of the granulosa cells during follicular development. If follicular development proceeds too slowly there is a rise in mutations in surviving ova. Studies of the effect of maternal diets of different protein content show very clearly the increase in the proportion of defective ova produced before fertilization as the ovulation rate and rates of cell replication decline.

PROTEIN INTAKE AND THE FIRST DAYS AFTER FERTILIZATION

Animal experiments show that the hypothalamus is more sensitive to the protein content of diet than the ovaries, embryo or foetus. Nelson and Evans (1954) showed that a protein-free diet fed to rat dams from mating resulted in 90 to 100 per cent embryonic resorptions, the foetal deaths occurring in most cases in 9 or 10 days. Injection of oestrone (0.5µg) and progesterone (4mg) daily maintained pregnancy in 100 per cent of dams and the number of living young was close to normal, again suggesting that the effect of nutrient deficiencies is via the hormone balance. The dams suffered major losses of body weight. Similar results were reported in experiments by Callard & Leathem (1970). Kinzey and Srebnik (1963) maintained pregnancy in rats fed a protein-free diet by using exclusively the pituitary hormones FSH, LH and prolactin. The availability of amino acids for follicular development and for embryonic and foetal growth is controlled by the endocrine system. Whether or not the protein in a particular diet is adequate for reproduction depends primarily upon the reaction of the hypothalamus to blood amino acid concentrations and not upon any direct effect of amino acids on the reproductive process, although individual amino acid deficiencies by themselves are mutagenic in cell culture (Freed & Schatz, 1969; Schempp & Krone, 1979).

Several studies have reported on the effects in animals of dietary protein restriction shortly before fertilization on embryonic cell replication immediately after mating. Muñoz and Malavé (1979) of the Venezuelan Institute of Scientific Research reported on these effects in mated female mice. It is seen in Table 4.2 that the mice on the lower protein diet produced fewer ova. The number of corpora lutea indicates the ovulation rate which is seen to be reduced by lowering the protein content of the diet. The ova were counted and few were lost before counting. It made no difference to the ovulation rate whether the rat dams were on the low protein diet for 2 weeks or 4 weeks before mating. This points to the existence of a period of heightened susceptibility to a low protein diet in mice lasting not more than 14 days.

Muñoz and Malavé examined the number of cell divisions in fertilized ova which happened 48, 72 and 96 hours after mating in rat dams which had been fed a standard or low protein diet during the 14 days before mating as shown in Figures 4.9, 4.10 and 4.11. The low protein diet produced cells that replicated slowly in contrast to the standard diet which produced cells which replicated at the normal rate. There were, in effect, fast and slow replication lanes. The failure to proceed to first cleavage indicates a defective ovum and probably a defective hormonal profile during ovulatory maturation. A subsequent rate of cell division below normal indicates a slow-down in DNA synthesis and an increase in risk of low birthweight and malformation in survivors. It is seen in Figure 4.11 that 34 ova in the slow lane had not proceeded even to first cleavage at 96 hours after mating and were unfertilized or carried defects originating around meiosis I or II. At the same time 122 ova in the

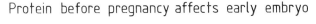

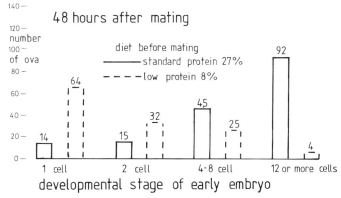

Figure 4.9. Fast and slow embryonic development in mice by maternal protein intake: at 48 hours. Source: Muñoz & Malavé, 1979, Table 3.

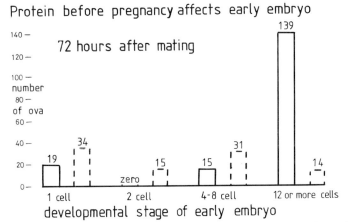

Figure 4.10. Fast and slow embryonic development in mice by maternal protein intake: at 72 hours. Source: Muñoz & Malavé, 1979, Table 3.

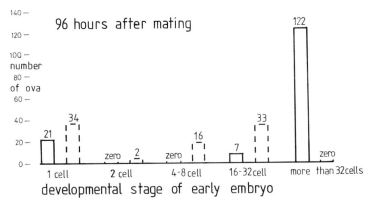

Figure 4.11. Fast and slow embryonic development in mice by maternal protein intake: at 96 hours. Source: Muñoz & Malavé, 1979, Table 3.

TABLE 4.2

EFFECT OF PROTEIN INTAKE ON NUMBER OF OVA AND NUMBER OF
CORPORA LUTEA IN MICE

percentage protein in diet	number of mice	average number per dam of	
		ova	corpora lutea
27	40	8.3 ± 0.9	8.85 ± 1.2
8	40	5.45 ± 1.0	5.6 ± 1.5

Source: Muñoz & Malavé, 1979.

fast lane had divided to produce embryos with 32 or more cells, but none of the ova from the dams on the low protein diet had reached this stage. Assuming all the ova in the slow lane were not defective the slow-down must have been a consequence of depressed levels of progesterone and possibly of other hormones. The unsatisfactory hormonal profile of the mice on the low protein diet prejudiced normal development before mating during ovulatory maturation, after ovulation and during fertilization and subsequently during the early stages of embryonic development. The low protein diet reduced fertility by causing fewer ova to be ovulated, caused damaged ova to be produced that did not survive and, by slowing down cell replication during the early stages of embryonic development, reduced the viability of any embryos that did in fact survive.

Mice have a high rate of metabolism and low nutrient reserves. Pigs in contrast have a much lower rate of metabolism and high nutrient reserves. Pond *et al.* (1968) of Cornell University showed that protein starvation of pigs instituted before breeding caused low or reduced fertility, low birthweight and stillbirth, in contrast to the slight effects of protein starvation during pregnancy. In pigs as in mice it is the protein status during the period immediately preceding mating that matters most.

The effects of a high as well as standard and low protein diet before mating on the reproduction of female mice have been reported by Tagami and Sudo (1982) working at the University of Ibaraki, Japan. The largest number of ova are seen in Figure 4.12 to have been produced by mice on a standard diet. Both low and high protein diets resulted in a lower ovulation rate. Mice are seen to be susceptible to percentages of protein in diet that are both too high and too low only one day before mating, a period which covers ovulatory maturation and meiosis I. Extension of the period on these diets before ovu-

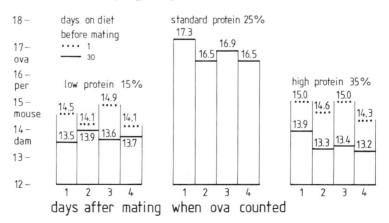

Figure 4.12. Modulation of ovulation rate in mice by protein intake.
Source: Tagami & Sudo, 1982, Table 1.

lation from 1 to 30 days had a further small but real effect on ovulation rate. It is shown in Figure 4.13 that the low and high protein diets also produced large numbers of abnormal ova. The classification of ova as abnormal by Tagami and Sudo would include the ova classified by Muñoz and Malavé as failing to proceed to first cleavage or subsequent failure to continue dividing. Studies by Tagami and colleagues have also shown that both abnormally high and low protein diets increase the length of the reproductive cycle, increase the time from introduction of the male to fertilization, increase the number of pups dying during lactation and reduce the growth rates of surviving pups.

It may be asked why then is too much protein harmful? Protein has to be metabolized and this requires enzymes. A high protein diet can produce competition for a coenzyme between the enzymes needed to metabolize surplus protein and enzymes needed for other purposes including growth and reproduction. Three coenzymes which have been shown to be a limiting growth factor in this way are riboflavin, pyridoxine and biotin. The endocrine system is sensitive to the blood serum concentrations of all these three nutrients.

The reaction of the endocrine system to maternal body weight and to total food intake and the effect on reproduction are discussed further in the next chapter.

Protein before pregnancy and percentage abnormal ova

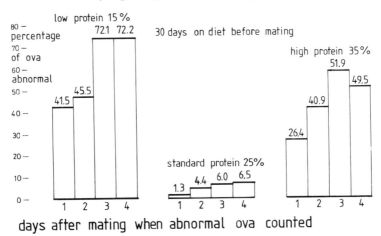

Figure 4.13. Abnormal ova produced by high and low protein intake in mice.
Source: Tagami & Sudo, 1982, Table 2.

THE EFFECT OF NUTRITION ON SPERMATOGENESIS

The testes like the ovaries are dependent for their function on the secretion of reproductive hormones by the hypothalamus and pituitary. As in the female the secretion of these hormones notably FSH and LH is modulated by nutrition. It has been shown that B vitamin deficiency causes infertility and atrophy of the testes in male animals which can be corrected by administration of pituitary hormones or the testicular hormone testosterone (Mann & Lutwak-Mann, 1981). However it is difficult, as in the female, to separate the direct effects of nutrient deficiency on the male testicular function and the indirect effects mediated by the hypothalamus and pituitary. A study of underfeeding male rats concluded that 'the basic problem in underfed rats is one of pituitary failure' (Howland, 1975). Deficiencies of vitamin A and zinc are examples of deficiencies that reduce the response of the cells of the testes to stimulation by testosterone. However vitamin A deficiency also disturbs the secretion of FSH by the pituitary (Huang *et al.*, 1983), and the uptake of zinc by the prostate is dependent on pituitary hormones (Gunn & Gould, 1957; Millar *et al.*, 1957).

When is spermatogenesis most susceptible to nutritional deficiency? Animals, usually mice, are used extensively for testing chemicals for mutagenicity. Komatsu and a team from the University of Tokio and the Japanese National Cancer Center noted that many chemicals under test reduced the food intake. They therefore undertook an investigation using mice to see how far reduced food intake alone was responsible for the mutagenicity rather than the chemical under test. A summary of some of their results is shown in Figure 4.14 using morphological abnormality of sperm as the indicator. Komatsu and his colleagues concluded that reduction of food intake is in itself mutagenic and that 'chemicals that reduce food intake cannot be screened' using animals in this way. This team also answered the question about the comparative susceptibility of the different stages of spermatogenesis. They found that Type B spermatogonia and early spermatocytes were most susceptible to food restriction (Komatsu *et al.*, 1982). As might be expected from the discussion in Chapter

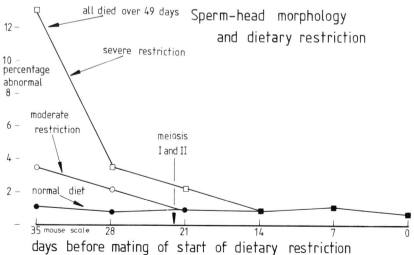

Figure 4.14. Increased sperm abnormalities in mice due to dietary restriction.
Source: Komatsu *et al.*, 1982, Figure 2.

Three illustrated in Figure 3.5 the highest susceptibility was during the time of maximum rates of DNA synthesis and cell replication.

Illness may cause men to go short of food for a week or a fortnight or longer. There is evidence that short term illness, such as appendicitis or ton-silitis, can cause important reductions in sperm concentration and motility, whether caused by the illness itself or short-term semi-starvation (David, 1982). A period of food restriction associated with illness is therefore a good reason for advising deferment of conception until Type B spermatogonia become available that were produced under conditions of health, that is 3 or 4 months from the return to health.

Low mineral content of semen is associated with male infertility, abnormal sperm morphology and low sperm motility as illustrated in Table 4.3 based on research by Pandy *et al.* (1983), of the Health Division of the Bombay Atomic Research Center.

TABLE 4.3

ASSOCIATION OF SPERM ABNORMALITY AND LOW SEMEN MINERAL CONTENT

	magnesium	calcium mg/dl	zinc
25 fertile men	14 to 18	24 to 28	19 to 24
23 infertile men	9.1	17.8	11.7
6 men with azoospermia	5.7	16.0	8.1
9 infertile men with worst sperm morphology	6.5	14.1	8.1
8 infertile men with lowest sperm motility	6.3	14.9	7.5

Source: Pandy *et al.*, 1983.

Deficiencies of magnesium and zinc have been shown to be mutagenic in animals and to cause chromosomal abnormalities as illustrated in Figure 4.15 (Bell *et al.*, 1975). Zinc deficiency has been shown to cause abnormal sperm morphology (Dinsdale & Williams, 1980). The association of infertility with low semen magnesium and zinc in Table 4.3 is not therefore unexpected, but cause and effect cannot be assumed because the men with low intakes of these particular minerals may have had low intakes of other nutrients. Low semen concentrations may also have causes other than low intake including malab-sorption and high excretion. Low semen mineral content is nevertheless a useful indicator of possible impaired fertility and of possible defective diet. Takahara *et al.* (1982) reported reduced fertility in male patients at seminal zinc levels below 15mg/dl and found zinc supplementation effective in im-proving fertility in 50 per cent of cases. The expediency of zinc supplemen-tation by itself without an investigation of diet must be doubted. Some of

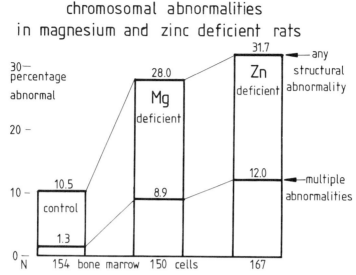

Figure 4.15. Mutation in maternal bone marrow in rats following mineral deficiencies.
Source: Bell *et al.*, 1975, Table 1.

Pandy's patients were deficient in magnesium not zinc and in others the effects of magnesium, zinc and calcium deficiency were probably additive.

The evidence is convincing that deficiencies of minerals other than magnesium and zinc can have serious effects on the fertility of farm animals. The correction of selenium deficiency is now established practice for animals grazing selenium deficient pastures. The most serious effect of selenium deficiency in domestic animals is on the fertility of the male (Wilkins & Kilgour, 1982). Bleau *et al.* (1984) of the University of Montreal have reported a significant correlation between sperm count and seminal selenium in man. Seminal selenium below 35ng/ml was found to be significantly associated with a low sperm count and a higher percentage of morphologically abnormal and non-viable sperm. The best pregnancy outcome in Bleau's series of 125 men consulting for infertility was associated with seminal selenium between 60 and 70ng/ml and fertile controls averaged 67.4 ± 5.4ng/ml. High intakes of selenium are toxic and mutagenic. The US National Research Council recommends a daily adult selenium intake between 50 and 200mcg. The expediency of selenium supplements that ignore the magnesium, zinc and other minerals is however doubtful. If data on actual deficiencies are not available, and it is thought that supplementation is desirable, it is difficult to justify any but balanced supplements. However deficiencies are not confined to minerals.

The effects of vitamin A deficiency on the fertility of male animals has been a subject of research since 1933 (Mason, 1933). Vitamin A deficiency in animals causes morphological abnormality of sperm and if prolonged causes complete disintegration and disappearance of spermatids and spermatozoa and nearly all spermatocytes (Mitranond *et al.*, 1979). Vitamin A is essential for DNA and RNA synthesis and for all cell replication (Omori & Chytil, 1982). Deficiency only appears to affect dividing spermatogonia, and the dormant, infrequently dividing, A_o spermatogonia appear in animal studies to be unaffected and able to regenerate cells, thus reviving spermatogenesis on restoration of vitamin A supply. Animal experiments throw doubts on the assumption that stores of vitamin A can be released quickly enough to protect germ cells if there is a sudden drop in intake. Some damage to sperm of male rats can be seen after exposure to a vitamin A deficient diet for only 72 hours in animals with adequate vitamin A stores (Kalla, 1981). Huang and Marshall (1983) stress that spermatogenesis in animals 'is extremely sensitive to changes in serum vitamin A levels'. It is nevertheless quite unclear whether or not the vitamin A deficiencies found in minorities of men in the western world are such as to interfere with spermatogenesis. The extensive research has been largely confined to animals and few research papers have been found that mention effects on men or women.

This chapter began with a discussion of the effects on reproduction, including spermatogenesis, of deficiencies of folic acid and cobalamin. Folic acid is one of the few nutrients for which there is both some information on the serum levels likely to affect spermatogenesis and on the prevalence of low serum levels in some populations. Thus a Canadian national survey found 11.2 per cent of Canadian men in the 20 to 39 age range to be at 'high risk' with serum levels of folic acid below 2.5ng/ml which is inadequate to maintain the intracellular levels needed for efficient DNA synthesis (Canada, 1975).

In animal husbandry male animals used for breeding are valuable and their feeding receives great care because any degree of infertility is expensive. As a single bull may have 20,000 offspring fertility may be measured in births as a percentage of inseminations, for which his owner is paid. The fertility of different bulls is found to vary from under 20 per cent to over 80 per cent which is close to the upper limit imposed by average fertility of the cows. There is a substantial and growing veterinary literature on bulls, rams, goatbucks, stallions, male mink, lions and other zoo animals showing that the right diet improves male reproductive performance and suggesting what is best. Mann and Lutwak-Mann (1981) in their treatise on 'Male Reproductive Function and Semen' say:

'There is hardly any component of ordinary diet that could be pronounced as unimportant to male reproductive function...'

The attitude to the nutrition of valuable male animals used for breeding is to reduce risks to a minimum. This requires supplementation if there is any doubt about adequacy of the diet for such minerals as zinc, selenium, iodine or vitamin A. Excessive intakes of some essential nutrients including zinc, selenium, manganese, iodine and vitamin A can increase mutation rate in animals and so increase risks and it is not therefore usual practice to supplement with more than reasonable physiological amounts of any nutrient.

Chapter Five includes a discussion of what are reasonable, desirable intakes of nutrients.

5. When does a woman's diet affect the outcome of her pregnancy?

OPTIMUM BIRTHWEIGHT AND MATERNAL NUTRITION

If a group of women is found to have babies in the optimum birthweight range it may be assumed that their diet was compatible with this happy outcome of pregnancy. The birthweight range associated with the lowest perinatal mortalities may be called the optimum birthweight range. This range is associated with the lowest incidence of birth defects as illustrated in Figure 5.1, which shows the incidence of perinatal deaths attributed to congenital anomalies for England and Wales. In the official statistics of several countries this optimum birthweight range with lowest mortalities is 3,500 to 4,500g, including the USA (US National Center for Health Statistics, 1972); Germany (Beck *et al.*, 1978); Scotland (Scottish Health Service, 1977); and Sweden (Sveriges Officiella Statistik, 1979). The optimum birthweight range in the official statistics of England and Wales is 3,500 to 4,000g, but figures for the range 4,000 to 4,500g are not published. Moreover infant mortalities in all countries are also very highly correlated negatively with birthweight, the mortality increasing only slowly at birthweights below 3,500g, more rapidly below 3,000g and

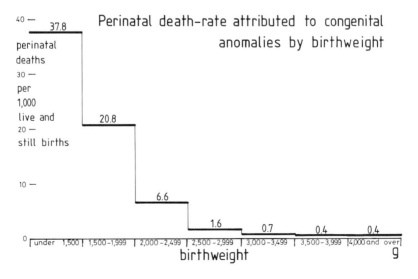

Figure 5.1. England and Wales. Source: OPCS, 1988.

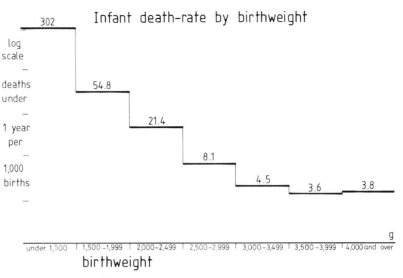

Figure 5.2. England and Wales. Source: OPCS, 1987.

more rapidly still below 2,500g. Figure 5.2 shows death-rates under 12 months of age by birthweight for England and Wales.

The diet eaten by 165 pregnant women whose babies were born into the optimum birthweight range was studied in a population of London women. Their nutrient intakes are set out in Table 5.1 with the diet of 28 mothers whose babies proved to be of low birthweight. The table is based on a study of diet in early pregnancy by Doyle *et al.* (1989b) of the Nuffield Institute of Comparative Medicine. The mothers were all patients at the Salvation Army Mothers' Hospital, Hackney, and in social class composition were approximately but not precisely representative of the British population, except that mothers of Asian origin were not included. Each mother kept a diary of food and drink for one week after interview and instruction. The diet was recorded in all cases around the end of the first trimester of pregnancy. The diet of the reference mothers in Table 5.1 is called the 'reference diet' and it is implied that it is a safe or desirable diet because shown to be compatible with a satisfactory birth outcome. The reference mothers are seen to have eaten more of all nutrients than the mothers of the low birthweight babies. For example the reference mothers consumed 74.5g/day average of protein while the mothers of the low birthweight babies consumed only 62.8g/day. Table 5.1 throws doubt on any suggestion that a protein intake below 75g/day is acceptable for women wishing to conceive or during pregnancy. This finding is in line with the old, but classical, papers of Bertha Burke and colleagues of the Harvard School of Public Health, published in the early 1940s, which showed associations of maternal protein consumption with birthweight and with birth length, illustrated in Figures 5.3 and 5.4. A low protein intake depresses gonadotrophin secretion, and for this reason alone the reduction of protein

TABLE 5.1

MEAN DAILY NUTRIENT INTAKES OF MOTHERS OF LOW BIRTHWEIGHT
BABIES ≤ 2,500g AND OF REFERENCE MOTHERS OF BABIES IN THE
OPTIMUM BIRTHWEIGHT RANGE 3,500 TO 4,500g; 193 LONDON MOTHERS

		n = 28	n = 165
birthweight range		≤ 2,500g	3,500–4,500g
energy	kcal	1,642	1,974
	MJ	6.87	8.26
protein	g	62.8	74.5
vitamins			
thiamin (B_1)	mg	1.0	1.2
riboflavin (B_2)	mg	1.5	2.0
niacin	mg	12.3	16.1
pyridoxine (B_6)	mg	1.2	1.5
folic acid	mcg	161	201
pantothenic acid	mg	3.7	4.4
minerals			
calcium	mg	761	953
iron	mg	9.4	12.9
magnesium	mg	209	283
phosphorus	mg	1,039	1,316
potassium	mg	2,493	2,993
sodium	mg	2,026	2,688
zinc	mg	8.16	10.2

Source: Doyle *et al.*, 1990

intake below 75g/day could be damaging to pregnancy outcome for some
women. However it was seen in the last chapter that maternal protein intake
begins to affect gonadotrophin secretion and pregnancy outcome already before pregnancy, during ovulatory maturation. The maternal protein intakes recorded by Burke and in the Hackney study during pregnancy were probably
similar to the intakes of the women's habitual diets and to their intakes around
the time of conception. Large trials of protein supplementation during the last
two trimesters of pregnancy have never produced increases in birth dimensions
in any way comparable to the differences in dimensions associated with differences in diet in the Hackney study (Rush, 1986). The extensively do-
cumented Women Infant and Child Supplemental Feeding Program (WIC) in
the USA showed little effect on birthweight or other pregnancy outcome (Rush
et al., 1988), except in one set of circumstances when mothers who had received extra food during one pregnancy continued to receive milk, cheese,

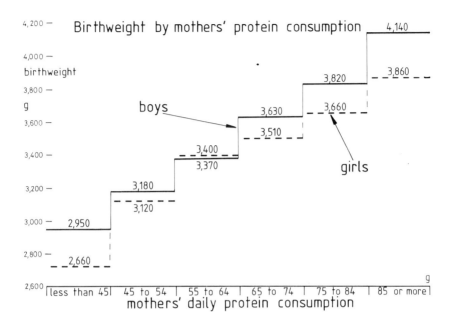

Figure 5.3. Harvard School of Public Health, 216 women.
Source: Burke *et al.*, 1943, Table VIII.

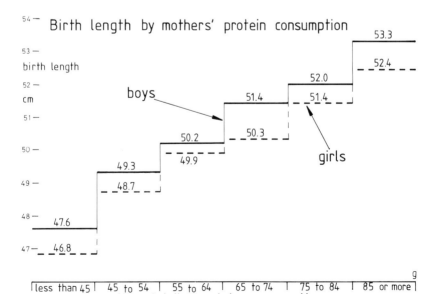

Figure 5.4. Harvard School of Public Health, 216 women.
Source: Burke *et al.*, 1943, Table VIII.

cereals, eggs and fruit juices during the subsequent interpregnancy interval and during the early months of the next pregnancy. The babies of the second pregnancy then had a significantly higher birthweight, birth length and a reduced risk of low birthweight (Caan *et al.*, 1987).

Maternal protein intake is invariably correlated with the intake of other nutrients and the associations in Figures 5.3 and 5.4. may have been wholly or partly caused by these other nutrients (Hurley, 1979). The Hackney study had a total of some 100,000 items of information and analysed not only the association of food and nutrient intake with birthweight but also with newborn length, head circumference, weight of placenta and length of gestation.

B VITAMINS AND BIRTH DIMENSIONS

Birth dimensions were found to be more significantly associated with maternal consumption of some B vitamins and with some minerals, notably magnesium, than with protein or calorie consumption. B vitamins are discussed first. Of all the constituents of maternal diet in the Hackney study B vitamins were most closely correlated with birth dimensions. Figure 5.5 shows the association of low birthweight with maternal intake of 4 B vitamins. The maternal intakes of thiamin and niacin were most closely correlated with birthweight, birth length and head circumference, with maternal intakes of riboflavin and pyridoxine next in significance. The hypothalamic pituitary-gonadal axis, as discussed in Chapter Four, is highly sensitive in other mammals to the intake of the B vitamins. Low intakes depressed gonadotrophin secretion and thereby follicular and embryonic development before there is any direct effect on germ or embryonic cells. The low intakes of B vitamins of the mothers at highest risk of a low birthweight baby, seen in Figure 5.5, may well have been associated with depressed levels of pituitary hormones which would increase the risk of low birthweight by slowing down ovulatory maturation before conception. In the Hackney study protein intake was also correlated with birth dimensions but at a lower level of significance than thiamin or niacin intakes and the correlations of maternal protein intakes with birth length and head circumference were only just significant ($p = 0.012$ & $p = 0.019$). This does not indicate that protein is unimportant for birth outcome but would be explained if there were many more Hackney women with B vitamin intakes than protein intakes low enough to depress pituitary hormone levels.

Studies of diets even in the most prosperous countries show that important minorities of women have daily intakes of B vitamins below recommended levels and have enzyme saturation levels involving 'moderate' or 'high' risk. Thus the Swiss 'Basle Study' of 6,400 employed adults found 22.8 per cent of women with depressed enzyme saturation for thiamin, 7.5 per cent for riboflavin, 25.9 per cent for pyridoxine (Ritzel, 1975). Another study of 200 pregnant women attending the Basel University Women's Clinic found 33 per

Probability of birthweight below 2500g by maternal intake of 4 B vitamins

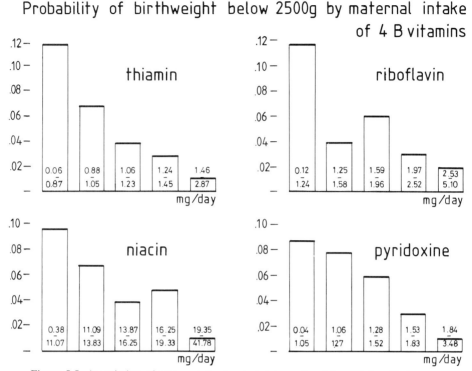

Figure 5.5. Association of maternal B vitamin intake and weight of baby. Hackney, London, 513 women. Source: Wynn *et al.*, 1991, Figure 6.

cent with depressed enzyme saturation for thiamin, 37 per cent for riboflavin and 27 per cent for pyridoxine (Decker *et al.*, 1975). A paper from the University of Kiel reported a significant correlation of low birthweight and low maternal thiamin intake in the first trimester, and referred to the 'surprisingly high proportion' of 229 women from 6 German teaching hospitals whose thiamin intake was inadequate to ensure an acceptable level of enzyme saturation (Kübler & Moch, 1975). The German Ministry of Youth, Family and Health sponsored a study by the University of Heidelberg into the nutrition of young men and women 20 to 40 years of age, and 621 women participated. The report commented particularly on thiamin intakes of both men and women and said (Arab *et al.*, 1982):

> 'Concurrently, in both sexes approximately 5 per cent show enzyme activation levels of transketolase that indicate extremely low coenzyme status, and another 25 per cent with borderline deficiency levels. The mean levels are comparable to those reported in the Swiss study of the Basel population but the prevalence of low levels is much greater in Heidelberg.'

Dividing cells have much higher energy requirements than cells that are not dividing. Ovulatory maturation and embryonic development involve the highest rates of cell replication in the human life cycle and therefore a high local availability of intracellular energy. DNA and RNA and protein synthesis require energy. Thiamin is an essential coenzyme for 3 enzymes concerned with the release of intracellular energy by the oxidation of glucose. Research on wound repair and scar development has shown that enzyme saturation with thiamin can be the factor limiting DNA and protein synthesis (Alvarez & Gilbreath, 1982; Im *et al.*, 1975). It would not therefore be surprising to find that low levels of enzyme saturation with thiamin might limit birthweight. In the volume on the American Recommended Dietary Allowances (US National Academy of Sciences, 1980) it is explained that the RDAs for thiamin of 1.1mg/day for women aged 19 to 22, and 1.0mg/day aged 23–50, were not adequate for enzyme saturation which indeed required a much higher intake. Because quite low levels of enzyme saturation are adequate for most body cells it does not follow, as assumed in the conception of the RDAs, that the rapid cell replication involved in the early stages of reproduction does not benefit from 100 per cent enzyme saturation. The average intake of thiamin of the reference women in Table 5.1 is seen to have been 1.2mg/day and of the mothers of the low birth-weight babies only 1.0mg/day, an intake close to the RDA of 1.0mg/day. Figure 5.5 shows that the risk of a low birthweight baby being born apparently decreased at least up to maternal intake levels of 1.46mg/day. The American RDAs for B vitamins may be satisfactory for women not intending to reproduce, but the maternal intakes in Figures 5.5 suggest that they are too low during the period preceding pregnancy or during pregnancy. The RDAs for pregnancy are increased to 1.4mg/day for thiamin, 1.5mg/day for riboflavin, 15mg/day for niacin, and 2.6mg/day for pyridoxine, but these higher levels, if they were followed, would only take effect after any deficiency had already caused an irreversible slow-down in follicular or embryonic development and after the placenta had developed to protect the foetus.

Nutritional deficiencies have their effects partly by their direct influence on the gonads and embryo and partly by their effect on the endocrine system. In other mammals the hypothalamus is more sensitive to a deficiency of thiamin than are the gonads or embryo. It is likely therefore that the associations found in the Hackney study and illustrated in Figure 5.5 were a consequence of depression of the hypothalamic-pituitary-ovarian axis. The hypothalamus in other mammals reacts to a severe deficiency of any of these B vitamins by inhibiting gonadotrophin secretion and so causing infertility (Watteville *et al.*, 1954). This reaction to an unsatisfactory diet, including a diet deficient in B vitamins, must have had survival value by inhibiting reproduction at times when fresh food was in short supply. However this depression of gonadotro-phin secretion is not a simple on-off mechanism and there is a penumbra between fertility and infertility illustrated in Figure 5.6. Within this penumbra hormonal and nutritional levels are not low enough to cause infertility but are still too low so that follicular growth is retarded, corpus lutea are too small and embryonic growth is retarded.

The Heidelberg report concluded that the greatest nutritional threat to women's health was too low a consumption of a number of nutrients notably thiamin, pyridoxine, folic acid, calcium and iron. The report said:

'Despite seemingly sufficient energy intakes, there is apparently an insufficient intake of some of the essential nutrients, particularly the B vitamins... The lower caloric needs of our passive society are met by lower intakes and when these are partially met by caloric sources which contribute few essential vitamins and minerals a deficiency is inevitable.'

Particularly before and around the time of conception a diet with a high density of B vitamins and essential minerals is desirable to maintain high levels of enzyme saturation.

Newborn head circumference in the Hackney study was significantly correlated with maternal intakes of thiamin and niacin ($p > 0.001$) as illustrated in Figures 5.7 and 5.8. The high statistical significance is largely attributable to the women who had babies with head circumferences below 34cm and particularly below 33cm. The average thiamin intake of the reference women in Table 5.1 was 1.2mg/day. This figure was only an average and made no allowance for variations in the requirements of individual women. As recommendation 1.2mg/day would have no safety margin to allow for individual variations and it is seen in Figure 5.5 that the risk of low birthweight continues to decline up to intakes of 1.46mg/day. The mothers of the babies with the largest birth head circumference in Figure 5.7 had an average thiamin intake of 1.28mg/day. Both Figures 5.5 and 5.7 suggest that thiamin intakes higher than 1.2mg/day may be desirable for some women. Animal experiments show that the efficiency of energy utilization increases with thiamin intake with rapidly diminishing, but nevertheless real, returns up to 2 or 3 times normal intake. The thiamin intake of the reference women of 1.2mg/day is the lowest

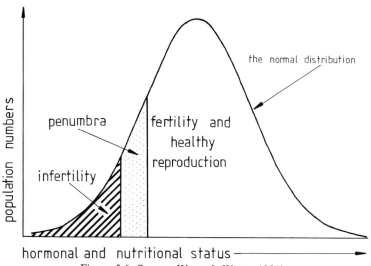

Figure 5.6. Source: Wynn & Wynn, 1981b.

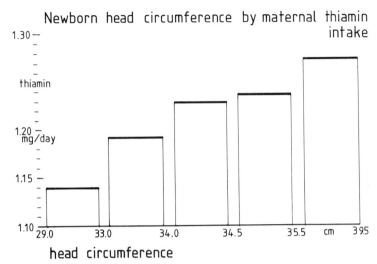

Figure 5.7. Association of maternal thiamin intake and head circumference of baby, Hackney, London, 513 women. Source: Doyle W. Personal communication.

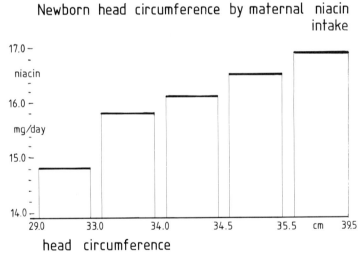

Figure 5.8. Association of maternal niacin intake and head circumference of baby, Hackney, London, 513 women. Source: Doyle, W. personal communication.

intake that can be regarded as acceptable for women anticipating pregnancy, but intakes up to 2mg/day may be desirable for some women. Similarly the niacin intake of the reference women was 16.1mg/day which may be regarded as the minimum desirable intake of women anticipating pregnancy, but Figure 5.5 suggests that some women may benefit from intakes over 19mg/day. Intakes of niacin up to 25mg/day may be necessary to allow for variations between women. Individual requirements depend on many factors and in particular on total energy requirements.

MAGNESIUM, AND OTHER ESSENTIAL MINERALS AND BIRTH DIMENSIONS

The placenta can extract vitamins from the mother's blood and transfer them at higher concentration to the foetus. The vitamin concentration in cord blood may be 5 or 10 times the concentration in maternal blood. This capacity of the placenta is sometimes referred to as the vitamin pump. There is no similar placental pump for minerals. The concentrations of minerals in maternal and foetal blood are compared in Table 5.2 and the differences are seen to be very small, in most cases statistically non-significant, and in no way comparable to the large differences often reported for vitamins (Gontzea, 1965; Hamfelt & Tuvemo, 1972; Van den Berg *et al.*, 1978). The foetus is not well-protected by the placenta from low mineral concentrations in maternal blood.

TABLE 5.2

SIMILARITY OF LEVELS OF MINERALS IN MATERNAL AND CORD
WHOLE BLOOD; 25 NORMAL BIRTHS, OXFORD, ENGLAND

| | mcg/ml | | | |
| | maternal | | cord | |
	mean	s.d.	mean	s.d.
iron	442	25	433	30
calcium	60	6	61	6
magnesium	36.2	3.9	36.7	3.4
zinc	7.7	1.1	7.6	0.7
copper	1.04	0.17	0.94	0.13
selenium	0.098	0.013	0.099	0.011
iodine	0.036	0.009	0.038	0.012
cobalt	0.021	0.007	0.024	0.005
manganese	0.012	0.005	0.015	0.007
chromium	0.007	0.003	0.009	0.005

Source: Bryce-Smith, 1985

In the Hackney study 54 out of 513 babies were born before 37 weeks' gestation (Doyle *et al.*, 1989a). The mineral intakes of the mothers of these

54 preterm babies are compared in Table 5.3 with the intakes of the mothers of babies born after 37 weeks gestation. There were no significant associations of preterm birth with maternal energy or protein intake or with intake of any vitamin except thiamin. Length of gestation is, however, difficult to record accurately and it is likely that the lower significance of the correlations of nutrient intakes with length of gestation compared with birthweight is partly a consequence of errors in recording.

The close association of maternal mineral intake and birthweight are shown in Table 5.4 for the mothers with babies of less than median birthweight. The

TABLE 5.3

THE MEDIAN MINERAL INTAKES OF MOTHERS OF BABIES BORN PRETERM BEFORE 37 WEEKS OR AFTER 37 WEEKS' GESTATION RANKED BY STATISTICAL SIGNIFICANCE OF DIFFERENCE; 513 LONDON MOTHERS

	n = 54 mg/day	n = 459 mg/day	p
magnesium	227	259	0.005
sodium	2268	2566	0.006
chlorine	3624	4016	0.008
iron	10.4	11.7	0.010
calcium	805	889	0.020
copper	1.42	1.51	0.020
phosphorus	1120	1244	0.021

Source: Doyle *et al.*, 1989a

TABLE 5.4

CORRELATIONS OF BIRTHWEIGHT WITH MATERNAL MINERAL INTAKES OF MOTHERS WITH BABIES BELOW THE MEDIAN BIRTHWEIGHT OF 3,270g; 255 LONDON MOTHERS

	correlation	
	r	p
magnesium	0.253	<0.001
iron	0.247	<0.001
phosphorus	0.243	<0.001
chlorine	0.240	<0.001
zinc	0.238	<0.001
sodium	0.237	<0.001
potassium	0.208	<0.001
calcium	0.184	0.002

Source: Doyle *et al.*, 1990

highest correlation is again seen to be with magnesium. None of the correlations for the same minerals were statistically significant for the mothers of babies of birthweight above the median of 3,270g.

The probability of birthweight being less than 3,000g by maternal magnesium intake is illustrated in Figure 5.9. The association of low birthweight and low maternal magnesium intake has been the subject of studies from a number of countries with some indication that it is the commonest mineral deficiency in many populations (Wynn & Wynn, 1988b). Trials of magnesium supplementation of women during pregnancy have reported significant reductions in the incidence of low birthweight and preterm birth (Spätling & Spätling, 1988). Magnesium is another nutrient essential for intracellular energy metabolism and participates in the same chemical reactions as thiamin. Deficiency of magnesium depresses the level of thiamin in body tissues as illustrated in Figures 5.10 from animal experiments (Itokawa *et al.*, 1973, 1974; Wynn & Wynn, 1988b). Thiamin cannot be used and is excreted if magnesium is deficient, with associated depression of intracellular energy metabolism. Magnesium is an essential cofactor for over 300 known enzymes, a much larger number than have been shown to require thiamin. It was noted in the last chapter that magnesium deficiency is mutagenic.

However maternal magnesium intake, and the maternal intake of all the other minerals in Table 5.4, were only associated with birthweight in the lower half of the birthweight range. This is illustrated in Figure 5.11 showing two cumulative average curves. These curves illustrate the important finding of the Hackney studies that the significant associations of maternal intakes of all nutrients and birth dimensions were limited to mothers of the smaller babies. In Figure 5.11 the cumulative average curve beginning from low birthweights falls to around 62 per cent of the reference diet value at birthweight around 2,000g, but rises to around the reference diet value somewhat below the me-

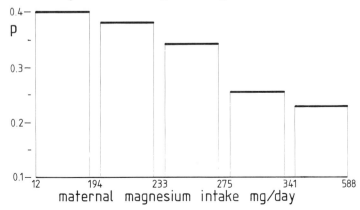

Figure 5.9. Association of maternal magnesium intake and birthweight 3,000g or less.
Source: Doyle *et al.*, 1989a, Figure 1.

dian birthweight of 3,270g. There is a plateau at higher birthweights indicating no significant association between birthweight and magnesium intake. The statistical significance of the difference between the two cumulative average curves may be computed for any birthweight and is found to be significant only below the median birthweight. This is an important conclusion because it follows that any major influence of nutritional deficiency in causing reduced birth dimensions must have been confined to a minority of mothers with the smaller babies.

Effect of magnesium deficiency on thiamin levels in rats

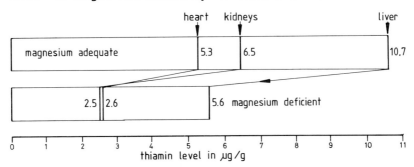

Figure 5.10. Depression of thiamin in tissues by magnesium deficiency. Sources: Itokawa *et al.*, 1974, Table 2; Wynn & Wynn 1988b, Figure 12.

Cumulative averages of maternal daily intakes of magnesium

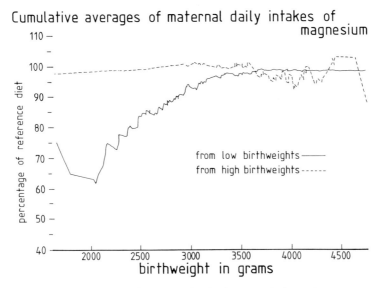

Figure 5.11. Low maternal magnesium intake in the lower half of the birthweight range. Source: Doyle *et al.*, 1989b, Figure 2.

WHEN DO NUTRITIONAL DEFICIENCIES HAVE THEIR EFFECTS?

There are several streams of evidence suggesting that the highest susceptibility to nutrient deficiency in the female is during ovulatory maturation and early embryonic development. Animal experiments show that deficiencies of some nutrients depress hormone levels and can cause infertility by preventing ovulation as illustrated diagrammatically in Figure 5.6. Lesser degrees of nutritional deficiency and depression of the hormonal status can cause delayed ovulation, reduced rates of early cleavage, low birthweight and congenital malformations in animals in the area described in Figure 5.6 as the penumbra. These results are produced before or around the time of mating. There is evidence that the supplementation of human pregnancy during the last two trimesters may benefit the mother and improve breast feeding but has very little effect on the foetus or pregnancy outcome, whereas the evidence of 50 years, from the Harvard studies of Burke to the London studies in Hackney of Doyle, show highly significant correlations of maternal nutritional status and birth outcome, associations that can only have had their origin very early in pregnancy. In the Hackney study vitamin and mineral supplements during the last two trimesters of pregnancy produced no significant effect on birth dimensions of the babies. In contrast vitamin supplements given before and around the time of conception in the trials of Smithells and colleagues in Leeds produced significant reductions in the risk of repetition of neural tube defects (Smithells *et al.*, 1983).

There is a long historical record from famines and during wars and the aftermath of wars showing the effect of food shortage on pregnancy outcome (Wynn & Wynn 1979, 1981b, 1981c). Many epidemics of perinatal mortality and congenital malformations were recorded following these periods of food shortage. The malformations such as neural tube defects are known to be of early pregnancy origin. The epidemic in Holland of congenital malformations following the 'hunger winter' of 1944–5 is illustrated in Figure 5.12. It is seen that the highest incidence of deaths caused by malformations was among babies conceived during the food shortage or during the following 4 months. The most serious consequences followed when the food shortage was before and around the time of conception. If a woman was short of food before or around the time that she conceived the risks to her baby were much more serious than if she was well fed at conception but short of food during pregnancy. The Dutch experience was repeated in Germany and other European cities.

The Dutch hunger produced a fall in the birth-rate of about 50 per cent, caused in part by stillbirths and early miscarriages. Such food shortages are today only a memory in the western world but how far does individual anorexia still cause infertility? The long history of anorexia nervosa and its effect on fertility goes back to the 19th century and also throws light on the effects of malnutrition on pregnancy outcome. The urinary and plasma gonadotrophins

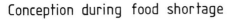

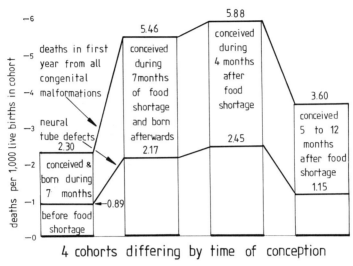

Figure 5.12. Epidemic of congenital malformations among babies conceived during and after the Dutch hunger winter 1944–45, 154, 365 births, 452 deaths. Sources: Stein *et al.*, 1975; Wynn & Wynn, 1987.

in anorexic, underweight women are low and may be too low to support follicular development and ovulation (Vigersky & Loriaux, 1977; Brown *et al.*, 1977). The hormones mainly affected are the pituitary hormones LH and FSH and the thyroid hormone T_3, and it is the resting level of LH that is particularly correlated with body weight independently of calorie intake. It is primarily failure of the LH surge to reach a critical level necessary for ovulation that causes infertility (Warren, 1977). Self-imposed weight loss by dieting has been shown to be a common cause of infertility and amenorrhoea of more than 50 per cent of women attending some infertility clinics (Nillius, 1978; Knuth *et al.*, 1977; Hirvonen, 1977; Bergh *et al.*, 1978). Nearly 80 per cent of infertile women have been judged to be underweight. What then is underweight in this context?

Women's weight is a rough indicator of nutritional status and its decline was recorded during the European food shortages by hospital clinics. There have been many subsequent studies in Europe and America showing the associations of fertility and pregnancy outcome with prepregnancy weight. These studies point again to the importance of nutritional status before conception. In a Swedish study the mean prepregnancy weight of 161 mothers of low birthweight babies was 53.9kg (Bjerre & Bjerre, 1976). The average Swedish women's body weight at the onset of amenorrhoea has been shown to be 52kg (Fries, 1974). The mothers of the low birthweight babies had, therefore, prepregnancy weight only 1.9kg above the infertility threshold for Swedish women. The average prepregnancy weight of Swedish women is 62.4kg, 8.5kg higher than the mothers of the low birthweight babies. Of the 161 low birth-weight babies in this study 28 died, 14 had congenital malformations or cere-bral palsy and 10 had minimal brain dysfunction at age 5. These were penumbral children.

Drugs may be used to induce ovulation. However a study in London teach-ing hospitals showed that amenorrhoeic women had a 25 per cent risk of having a small-for-dates, growth retarded baby following induced ovulation, and this risk increased to 54 per cent if the women were underweight (van der Spuy *et al.*, 1988). This important study extended to women the findings of Kinzey and Srebnik (1963) who showed that the maintenance of pregnancy with estrone and progesterone in protein deficient animals produced low birth-weight offspring.

Prepregnancy maternal weight was highly correlated with birthweight in the Hackney study, with a correlation coefficient of 0.235 (Doyle *et al.*, 1989b). This compares with correlation coefficients of 0.260 for pregnancies of Ameri-can black mothers and 0.290 for white mothers in the US Collaborative Peri-natal Study (Niswander & Jackson, 1974). The percentages of low birthweight babies among 7,054 American white women and 8,175 black women in the Collaborative Study are shown in Figure 5.13 for different prepregnancy weights. The association with height is eliminated in this figure by selecting only women in the height range 160 to 165cm (Niswander & Gordon, 1972). The 165 Hackney reference mothers had an average weight of 63kg (10 stone 9 lbs) a figure close to the average for Swedish women of 62.4kg.

Surveys over many years have shown an association between maternal height, birthweight and perinatal mortality. The Hackney study found a signi-

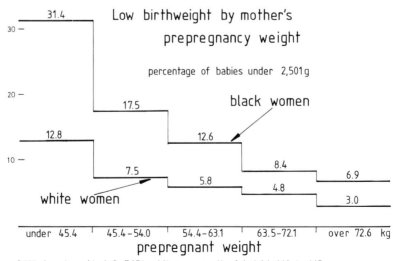

Figure 5.13. The association of low prepregnancy weight and low birthweight independently of height. Source: Niswander & Gordon, 1972, Chapter 7 Section 2.

ficant association between maternal height and nutrient intake, shown in Table 5.5. Maternal shortness was a risk factor associated with eating less of a poorer quality diet and a poorer social background. Prepregnancy weight is however in all surveys much more closely associated with birthweight and other birth dimensions than is prepregnancy height and the Hackney study found no correlation between social class and prepregnancy weight.

TABLE 5.5

CORRELATION OF MATERNAL HEIGHT AND MATERNAL NUTRIENT INTAKES WITH SIGNIFICANCE BETTER THAN p = 0.01; 513 LONDON WOMEN

	r	p
fibre	0.162	<0.001
magnesium	0.145	<0.001
niacin	0.137	<0.001
folic acid	0.136	<0.001
thiamin	0.127	0.002
fat	0.121	0.003
phosphorus	0.120	0.003
pyridoxine	0.119	0.003
energy	0.112	0.006
social class	0.188	<0.001

Source: Doyle W., personal communication.

Maternal height may be taken into account by using the body mass index (BMI) (weight in kilograms divided by height in metres squared kg/m^2). The 165 Hackney reference women who had babies within the optimum weight range had a BMI of $23.7kg/m^2$. This is close to the average for American women of reproductive age of $24.0kg/m^2$. The BMI is easy to assess and the figure of $24.0kg/m^2$ may be regarded as a satisfactory value for women anticipating pregnancy. Prepregnancy weight is a risk factor with risk increasing as the BMI falls below $24kg/m^2$. The American infertility threshold is reported to be $20.8kg/m^2$ for 50 per cent fertility (Frisch, 1977), with only 10 per cent fertility at $18.2kg/m^2$. There is nothing inevitable about an unfavourable outcome of the pregnancy of the low weight mother, nor does an ample prepregnancy weight eliminate all risk. There are other risk factors such as low B vitamin, magnesium or iron intakes. Effective action to reduce these risks is possible. This can be better understood from the systematic studies in animal husbandry.

In reacting to body weight the hypothalamus is reacting to past nutrition over a period of weeks and months. One problem in animal husbandry is deciding how long the period of nutritional preparation between pregnancies should be. Failed insemination particularly in cattle is expensive not only because artificial insemination has to be paid for but because it increases the period of unproductive maintenance. All mammals have an infertility threshold and both long and short term effects are described in the extensive literature of animal husbandry. For example the farming practice of 'flushing' has been defined in the context of sheep farming (Coop, 1966):

'The practice of giving ewes which are in fairly poor condition an improved diet for a few weeks before mating so that they are in a rapidly rising condition when they meet the ram.'

Ovulation rate and numbers of surviving young depend on the nutritional status of cows, ewes and other domestic animals and in particular on energy balance before mating (Haresign & Cole, 1981). However a longer term effect of poor nutrition can only be partly overcome by flushing. Low body weight in animals is almost synonymous with 'poor condition', but flushing is not just a matter of fattening but of supplying all those nutrients, provided for example by fresh pasture, which are needed by the hypothalamus and pituitary to provide an excellent hormonal profile.

There are, indeed, long and short term effects of diet on fertility and pregnancy outcome. The effects of a less than adequate diet, if it has not been too inadequate, can be offset by an excellent diet for a few weeks before and around conception.

APPETITE AND EXERCISE

A recommendation that anyone should consume a better diet may be defeated by lack of appetite. Anorexia nervosa cannot be cured simply by advising the sufferer to eat more. Loss of appetite is an important clinical sign but difficult to interpret. It is common in most diseases involving the digestive system. Poor appetite is, however, a problem of important minorities in developed countries who have no diagnosable digestive illness.

In the Hackney study the majority of low birthweight babies were born to a minority of women with abnormally low energy intakes and low intakes of other nutrients. The case histories of many of these mothers reported a 'poor appetite'. Of 1,582 pregnant women attending the Montreal Diet Dispensary 19.7 per cent had an intake below 1,719 kcal/day and 9.8 per cent below 1,453 kcal/day at first attendance and many of these women had poor appetites. A Canadian national survey showed that 25 per cent of pregnant women were consuming less than 1,655 kilocalories (Canada, 1975). American surveys show that, taking only women with incomes above the poverty level, there are substantial minorities with very low calorie intakes (US National Center for Health Statistics, 1979).

Appetite is psychosomatic and the somatic component includes the effect on appetite of the food actually consumed. Appetite grows by what it feeds on. Poor quality diet can cause both conscious and unconscious loss of appetite. Thiamin deficiency causes loss of appetite which has been described as 'more specific and severe' than the loss of appetite caused by deficiencies of other vitamins or of amino acids (Gubler, 1982). Deficiencies of riboflavin, niacin, pyridoxine, folic acid, biotin and vitamin C have been reported to depress appetite. Deficiencies of minerals including magnesium, phosphorus, sodium and zinc depress appetite as also do excesses of calcium, iron, manganese and sodium (Werbach, 1988; Trémolière, 1977).

What is eaten depends on appetite to the extent that availability is under control. Nutritional requirements are increased by exercise which generally increases appetite. Experiments on athletes expending between 3,000 and 4,500 kilocalories a day found that they adapted their calorie food consumption with a time lag of about 2 days. They ate more or less according to their energy requirements hardly aware of their changes in appetite (Trémolière, 1977). Exercise in a female athlete can, however, result in amenorrhoea as a consequence of depression of the hypothalamic-pituitary-ovarian axis with the same effect on the axis as a poor diet. Amenorrhoea has been reported to affect 50 per cent of competitive runners, 44 per cent of ballet dancers, 25 per cent of non-competitive runners, 12 per cent of swimmers and cyclists (Calabrese *et al.*, 1983; Sanborn *et al.*, 1982). Amenorrhoea was for long considered to be a benign side effect of athletic training, but there is now evidence that the low levels of oestradiol with which it is associated produce lower bone density and predispose to osteoporosis (Nelson *et al.*, 1986). Comparison of two groups of eumenorrhoeic and amenorrhoeic women runners showed that the amenorrhoeic women had the lower average intakes of energy including carbohydrate, fat and protein. The study concluded that the amenorrhoea might be explained by inadequate diet, which would be expected to depress gonadotrophin secretion. Appetite alone does not ensure the consumption by some women athletes of a diet adequate to prevent amenorrhoea. Japanese studies have reported a serious aggravation of thiamin deficiency among poor male students from engaging in athletic pursuits (Hatanaka & Ueda, 1981). Riboflavin is another nutrient required in increased amount by women taking daily exercise. The present recommended dietary allowances in the U.K. and U.S.A. are borderline for the average sedentary woman, and riboflavin status rapidly deteriorates with moderate exercise such as jogging (Belko *et al.*, 1983). Riboflavin deficiency, as we have seen, also causes hormonal imbalance.

Appetite alone can result in too high as well as too low a consumption and depends in complicated ways on food composition and even on the order in which different foods are consumed. Appetite cannot be relied upon to ensure an optimum food intake and hormonal balance.

FOOD EATEN BY MOTHERS OF LOW AND OF OPTIMUM BIRTHWEIGHT BABIES

It was seen in Table 5.1 that the mothers of low birthweight babies in Hackney ate less on average than the mothers of babies of optimum birthweight; the reference mothers ate more of virtually every essential nutrient. The foods recorded in the diaries of the reference women were different also in quality. The difference is summarized using food groups in Table 5.6. The first food group in this table is breakfast cereals including muesli, oats, nuts and seeds. This food group had the highest density of B vitamins and contributed more than 20 per cent of thiamin and niacin to the total diet and was also responsible for around 40 per cent of the difference in the intakes of B vitamins between these two groups of mothers. This same food group also made a major contribution to the intake of magnesium and other minerals, and a 22 per cent contribution to the difference in energy intake between the two groups. This first group alone emphasizes the importance of breakfast. The next food group 'eggs and egg dishes' shows a difference of 121kJ between the two groups of women, a difference much greater than for bacon and ham which was only 19kJ and was included in the meat group at the bottom of the table. The maternal consumption of wholemeal bread is also seen to be associated with higher birthweight and of white bread with lower birthweight. The first three groups in the table appear to be relevant to the breakfast menu.

The next two groups 'sugar and jams', 'biscuits and cakes' contributed together a quarter of the difference in calorie intake between the two groups of mothers but only about 4 per cent of the difference in magnesium intake and less still for the intake of vitamins. The reference mothers are then seen to have had appreciably higher intakes of fats and of fish than the mothers of the low birthweight babies. However the next important difference between the two groups of mothers was in the consumption of dairy produce which was responsible for 28 per cent of the difference in energy intake and a similar percentage difference for many minerals such as calcium and magnesium and vitamins such as riboflavin.

'Vegetables' made a major contribution to B vitamin intake and to the maternal intake of important minerals including magnesium. Vegetables were, indeed, the most important contributor of magnesium with dairy produce in second place and were more important than dairy produce as a source of B vitamins.

TABLE 5.6

DIET BY MAJOR FOOD GROUPS OF MOTHERS OF LOW BIRTHWEIGHT
BABIES ≤ 2,500g AND OF REFERENCE MOTHERS WITH BABIES BORN
BETWEEN 3,500 AND 4,500g; 193 LONDON MOTHERS

food group	intake of foods in kilojoules/day		
	a mothers of babies ≤ 2,500g n = 28	b mothers of babies 3,500–4,500g n = 165	a as percentage of b
breakfast cereals, muesli, oats, nuts and seeds	339	632	53.6
eggs and egg dishes	179	300	59.7
wholemeal bread	128	203	63.1
sugar and jams	310	455	68.2
biscuits and cakes	515	722	71.3
fats (marg., butter, oils)	328	456	71.9
fish	138	187	73.9
dairy produce	1,348	1,732	77.8
fruit	280	351	79.7
vegetables	934	1,087	85.9
potatoes	644	703	91.5
meat products	469	468	100.2
white bread	620	598	103.6
meat	873	842	103.7
soft drinks	286	232	123.3
total	6,820	8,170	83.5

Source: Doyle *et al.*, 1990

It seen that meat, meat products, white bread and soft drinks were consumed in marginally greater average amounts by the mothers of the low birthweight babies. The hypothesis that an increased consumption of meat or of white bread or soft drinks would benefit pregnancy outcome was contradicted for this particular population. The hypothesis that the energy intake of the mothers of low birthweight babies was too low was not contradicted. The hypothesis that the diet of the mothers of low birthweight babies had too low a nutrient density is supported. The major difference between the diets of the two groups of women was in the intake of foods of high nutrient density, including breakfast cereals, muesli, oats, nuts, seeds, eggs, egg dishes, wholemeal bread, dairy produce, fruit and vegetables.

6. Mutagens and antimutagens

The opening chapter of this book asked what is the origin of genetic diseases that reduce fertility and so are not maintained by children inheriting from parental sufferers, but which nevertheless do not die out and sometimes increase in prevalence. We described these as one-generation genetic diseases. These diseases include Down's syndrome, a substantial part of all diabetes, epilepsy, fragile X syndrome and many kinds of mental and physical handicap. The risk of these diseases increases with parental mutation rates.

Most research on mutation is financed by cancer research funds but amongst the studies published are many describing mutation in germ cells and discussing environmental mutagens. Study has expanded to include antimutagens, which are substances that destroy mutagens or inhibit their effects. Diet may be more or less mutagenic, or, in the words of a study from Ames (1983): 'Diet is a source of mutagens and antimutagens'. Where are mutagens to be found and can they be avoided? Where are antimutagens to be found and are they a defence? A report from the International Commission says (ICPEMC, 1986):

> 'In view of the widespread occurrence of mutagenic compounds in food and beverages as well as in other parts of the environment, effective elimination of exposure to many genotoxic chemicals is not feasible.'

The report explains that it is not referring only to mutagenic chemicals in the environment of our industrial society such as lead or various constituents of smoke but also to the naturally occurring mutagens including oxygen radicals produced in food by oxidation for example of some fatty acids. In the context of reproduction a diet that is too mutagenic is a bad diet. The possibility of defence against the mutagens in the environment by antimutagens in food introduces a new scale of good and bad. The search for antimutagens is worldwide and expanding (Knudsen, 1986). The International Commission commented:

> 'One group of likely candidates for safe use in mutation and cancer prevention are natural constituents in our diet. These may at present actually determine the level of protection against genotoxic compounds. This applies to vitamins A, C and E and also to selenium in areas of low selenium intake.'

The intake of foods and drinks may be changed to increase the antimutagenicity of a daily diet. This is relevant to choice of diet during the days and weeks before and around conception when the risk is high of new mutations, which are almost invariably harmful. It was noted in Chapter Four that a deficiency of protein and of particular vitamins and minerals could increase mutation rate. The role of some nutrients like vitamins A, C and E and of minerals like selenium in making some mutagens less potent or harmless may be of consequence even when diets cannot be described as deficient. Mutagens and antimutagens can modulate mutagenicity whether or not a diet is adequate by conventional criteria. Apart from some vitamins and minerals the antimutagens chemically identified so far include many less familiar plant constituents notably phenolic compounds, including some tannins and flavonoids, ellagic acid and gallic acid, sulfhydryl compounds including glutathione, carotenes, some terpenes, indoles and cyanates (ICPEMC, 1986).

The present chapter discusses mutagens and antimutagens in diet within the digestive tract. Only the part of the diet absorbed makes a contribution to mutation rate and this contribution is very variable depending upon the contents of the digestive tract. Vitamins A, E, betacarotene and vitamin C which survive digestion and are absorbed continue their antioxidant role within the body. Among the important antimutagens within the body are the heme containing proteins which include the mutagen-metabolizing enzymes of the liver. These antimutagens contain iron which is best provided by heme in the diet. The antimutagenicity of heme is illustrated in Figure 6.1. Among the defences of every body cell against mutagens is the active enzyme glutathione peroxidase, which requires the essential nutrient selenium. A shortage of selenium can cause a raised mutation rate (Hayatsu *et al.*, 1988; ICPEMC, 1986). These endogenous antimutagens are synthesized within the body and their synthesis requires an efficient supply of all the essential nutrients needed for protein synthesis including efficient intracellular energy metabolism. There are, however, many antimutagens in food that are not classified as essential nutrients.

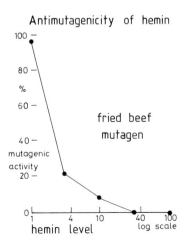

Figure 6.1. Source: Hayatsu *et al.*, 1981b, Figure 1.

THE ANTIMUTAGENICITY OF FRESH VEGETABLES AND FRUIT

Most of the known antimutagens are naturally occurring constituents of plants including familiar vegetables and fruits. Kada and his colleagues of the Department of Induced Mutation of the Japanese Institute of Genetics have made systematic searches for such constituents by measuring the inhibiting effect of plant juices on the mutagenic action in bacteria of the pyrolysis products of amino acids produced by, for example, cooking meat at excessively high temperatures (Kada *et al.*, 1978; Kada, 1982). The pyrolysis of protein produces a range of mutagens of great potency, many of which have now been chemically identified. Among the antimutagenic plant juices first identified were those of cabbage, ginger, radish and turnip. The results for cabbage juice are summarized in Table 6.1. The mutagen used in this study, Try-P, was produced by the pyrolysis of the amino acid tryptophan. It is seen in Table 6.1 that the antimutagens in cabbage were destroyed by boiling for 30 minutes, while the mutagen was not destroyed. The antimutagens in cabbage were not identified and were not in the cabbage fibre but in the juice and were not precipitated by a centrifuge. Many of the antimutagens in other vegetables are also destroyed by boiling.

TABLE 6.1

THE ANTIMUTAGENICITY OF CABBAGE JUICE AND ITS DESTRUCTION
BY BOILING; AMES TEST USING TRY-P AS MUTAGEN

treatment	mutations per plate
no cabbage juice, no mutagen	44
cabbage juice, but no mutagen	41
mutagen and raw cabbage juice	51
mutagen and boiled cabbage juice	280
mutagen only	295

Source: Kada *et al.*, 1978; Ames *et al.*, 1975

Fifty-nine different vegetables and fruits were examined by Morita *et al.* (1978), also from the Japanese Institute of Genetics, and they found that all except 2 were in some degree antimutagenic, again using mutagens produced by the heating of amino acids. Thirty-six of these vegetables and fruits are listed in Table 6.2 in order of their antimutagenicity against a single mutagen, again Try-P. Burdock (*arctium lappa*) at the top of the list is cultivated as a vegetable in Japan and young leaves, stems and roots are eaten. Taro (*Colocasia esculenta*) is a root vegetable of Asian origin with many varieties widely used in tropical countries. The full list in Morita's paper included other Japanese vegetables not sold by the British greengrocer, but none of great antimutagenic merit although some Japanese mushrooms are of interest. The ranking of fresh foods, as illustrated in Table 6.2, is different for other mut-

TABLE 6.2

THE COMPARATIVE ANTIMUTAGENICITY OF SOME FRESH FOODS;
PERCENTAGE OF MUTAGEN INACTIVATED

burdock	95	turnip leaf	55
mint leaf	93	taro	51
broccoli	91	garlic	48
green pepper	91	banana	47
apple	87	pears	46
shallot	87	mandarin oranges	42
pineapple	87	rape blossom	41
ginger	85	Chinese cabbage	35
cabbage	83	Welsh onion	34
aubergine	81	lettuce	29
beefsteak plant	78	pumpkin	29
parsley	78	celery	27
cauliflower	76	yam	23
grapes	74	turnip root	15
sweet potato	65	green asparagus	10
radish	59	red cabbage	8
chicory	58	cucumber	5
oranges	55	field pea	1

Source: Morita *et al.*, 1978.

agens and each antimutagen has its own spectrum. Some antimutagens have a wide spectrum and some a narrow. For example tested against the mutagenic pyrolysis products of 4 other amino acids burdock, broccoli and aubergine were found to be effective antimutagens for all 4, while apples were effective against 3 and cabbage against only one. The limited spectrum of most if not all antimutagens is a great complication and is characteristic not only of food extracts like apple juice but of chemical constituents like vitamin C.

Most of the new antimutagenic compounds currently being discovered are plant constituents, but many of the most effective are heat-labile and difficult to isolate and have been shown in particular cases to be specific proteins and enzymes. More than a 100 specific chemicals have been identified as anti-mutagens. The difficulty of deciding on any application of the research on antimutagens may be illustrated from the research on tea which is produced from the leaves of *camellia sinensis*. Over 70 per cent of the soluble matter in tea consists of tannins which are derivatives of the compound catechin. One particular catechin (epigallocatechin gallate) making up to 5 per cent of green tea powder has been found to be a very potent antimutagen (Kada *et al*, 1985). It is a long way from such a discovery to establishing the range of mutagens and biological environments in which green tea extracts are effective. However such a discovery is to be taken seriously because tea is used by around one half the world's population and catechins are reasonably stable compounds.

How far are the antimutagens in foods a defence against mutagens found in the environment? Nitroso compounds are an important class of mutagens that occur naturally, but have been increased in the human environment by pollution of water with nitrates from agricultural fertilizer and by some methods of food preservation used in the manufacture of ham and bacon, some other preserved meats, some kinds of cheese, smoked products and some cosmetics. Smoke including vehicle exhaust gases contains oxides of nitrogen that can be precursors of these mutagens. Two precursors of nitroso compounds were used as mutagens in experiments by Barale *et al.* (1983) of the University of Pisa. The antimutagenicity of carrots, cauliflower, lettuce, spinach and strawberries is illustrated in Figures 6.2 and 6.3 based on this research. Male mice were used in the experiments and yeast was used for measuring mutagenic activity. These experiments illustrate the antimutagenicity of some fresh foods for a particular class of mutagen. Figure 6.2 is based on measurements of mutagenicity of the contents of the digestive tract and shows the antimutagenicity of 5 juices. Many antimutagens act in this way, preventing the absorption of mutagens and also preventing mutation in the lining of the digestive tract. Figure 6.3 based on intrahepatic measurements shows that the 5 juices continued to be effective against nitroso compounds after absorption, but with a different order of antimutagenic potency. In both experiments juices

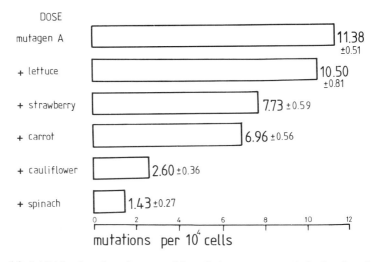

Figure 6.2. Inhibition in mice of mutagenicity of nitroso compounds in the digestive tract by fruit and vegetable juices. Source: Barale *et al.*, 1983, Table 1.

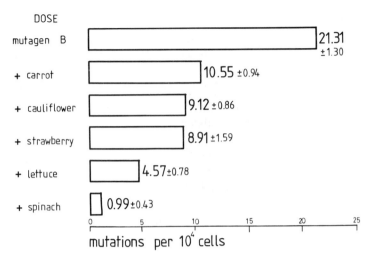

Figure 6.3. Inhibition in mice of mutagenicity of nitroso compounds in the liver by fruit and vegetable juices. Source: Barale *et al.*, 1983, Table 1.

were used and not whole vegetables so that the antimutagens must have been in the juices and not in the fibre.

Many mutagens cause mutations by reacting chemically with DNA for example by alkylation. Yano (1979) of Saitama Medical School, investigated the effect of the juice of 7 vegetables and milk on the mutagenicity of alkylating mutagens. The 7 vegetable juices decomposed these mutagens and made them non-mutagenic in different degrees as illustrated in Table 6.3. The potency of milk in inhibiting alkylation was greater than that of the vegetable juices on a volume basis. Milk has however a higher solid content than the vegetable juices, so Yano recalculated potency using an arbitrary scale based on freeze-dried material and it was then comparable with the fresh vegetable juices.

A growing list of desirable, but not essential, antimutagenic nutrients is being added to the lists of essential nutrients accepted as necessary for survival. Chlorophyll, the green colouring constituent of plants essential for photosynthesis, is an example of a desirable nutrient. It was reported in 1979 from the University of Texas that chlorophyll appeared to be the most active antimutagenic substance in wheat sprouts (Lai *et al*, 1980). It has been shown in many subsequent studies that chlorophyll, or its salt chlorophyllin, is an antimutagen with an exceptionally broad spectrum. Ong *et al.* (1986, 1989) of the US National Institute of Occupational Safety and Health compared the potency of chlorophyllin, retinol, beta-carotene, vitamin C and vitamin E as anti-mutagens. Figure 6.4 illustrates the antimutagenic effect of chlorophyllin on fried minced pork. Ong prepared other mixtures of mutagens from substances to which it was thought that many people are often exposed, including coal dust, diesel engine emission particles, airborne dust particles, tobacco

TABLE 6.3

COMPARATIVE ANTIMUTAGENIC POTENCY OF 8 FOODS IN DE-
STROYING ALKYLATING ACTIVITY OF N-METHYL-NITROSO UREA (MNU)

	percentage reduction in activity volume basis	effectiveness arbitrary scale dry basis
radish	40.3	20.4
cabbage	44.7	11.3
garden pea	77.8	10.7
lettuce	17.3	8.3
cucumber	26.0	7.9
celery	30.1	7.4
milk	80.4	7.2
tomato	44.1	7.0
water	0.0	0.0

Source: Yano, 1979

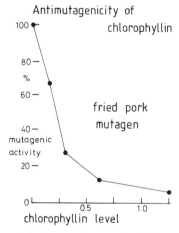

Figure 6.4. Source: Ong *et al.*, 1986, Table 1.

snuff and beef over-cooked at 230°C. Chlorophyllin was 69 per cent effective against the tobacco snuff and 90 per cent against the 4 other complex mixtures. Retinol was 29-48 per cent effective against all 5 mixtures, beta-carotene somewhat less so and vitamins C and E almost ineffective. Beta-carotene, although a precursor of retinol, is not itself an essential nutrient, but is an antimutagen and desirable nutrient that is entering large scale production by the drug industry in USA. The Ames test used by Ong can do no more than identify possibly useful substances and the paper concluded:

'It seems that chlorophyllin is potentially useful for the prevention of health hazards that may be caused by genotoxic agents.'

The antimutagenicity of chlorophyll may be another reason why it is wise to consume green vegetables, but assessment of the practical value of this knowledge remains to be done together with similar information about other antimutagens.

The B vitamins are important antimutagens. Benzpyrene is a mutagenic constituent of smoke and it is seen in Figure 6.5 based on Dutch research that riboflavin is an antimutagen for benzpyrene and also for cigarette smoke condensate (Terwel & van der Hoeven, 1985). B vitamins are essential for DNA synthesis and repair, and it has been shown, for example, that niacin reduces oxygen radical induced damage to DNA (Weitberg, 1989).

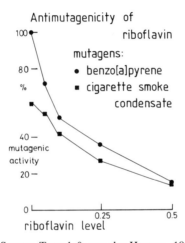

Figure 6.5. Source: Terwel & van der Hoeven, 1985, Figure 2.

THE ANTIMUTAGENICITY OF SOME FATS AND OILS

The overall mutagenic status of a diet depends on the potency and concentration of mutagens and antimutagens it contains. Unsaturated fatty acids provide an important part of the antimutagenicity of most diets. The most ubiquitous fatty acid with the highest concentration in most foods is oleic, which is monounsaturated. The antimutagenicity of oleic and other fatty acids has been studied by Hayatsu and colleagues of the Faculty of Pharmaceutical Sciences, Okayama University (Hayatsu *et al.*, 1981a, 1981b. 1988). The antimutagenicity of oleic acid is illustrated for one mutagen in Figure 6.6, but oleic acid is effective in the inhibition of a broad spectrum of mutagens including not only protein pyrolysis compounds, but nitroso compounds and polycyclic hydrocarbons.

Olive oil contains from 65 to 85 per cent of oleic acid and an average of 11 per cent of linoleic acid, the most ubiquitous polyunsaturated fatty acid

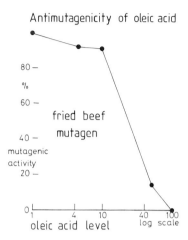

Figure 6.6. Source: Hayatsu *et al.*, 1981b, Figure 1.

which is an even more potent antimutagen than oleic. The potency of different vegetable oils as antimutagens varies widely, the most potent being safflower seed, sunflower seed, soyabean oil and corn oil in that order. Coconut or palm oil contain substantial percentages of saturated fatty acids which have no effect on mutagenic status. Of the grains oats has the highest percentage of unsaturated fatty acids, 16 per cent of its energy value depending on these unsaturated fats compared with less than 5 per cent for wheat. The antimutagenicity of some dozen unsaturated fatty acids has been studied and they have all been found to be antimutagenic in different degress. However Hayatsu (1981a, 1981b) reported that the ether extract of normal human faeces was antimutagenic and that oleic and linoleic acids were the effective inhibitors. The full significance of this finding is still not clear, but it seems that one role of these unsaturated fatty acids is the maintenance of the antimutagenicity of the whole contents of the digestive tract. New mutagens are generated during digestion so consumption of antimutagens is desirable apart from the need to neutralize mutagens in the diet. Meals based too heavily on some carbohydrates may contain too little unsaturated fat, although some whole grains notably oats contain adequate fat of excellent quality.

Any commendation of unsaturated fats for their antimutagenicity applies only to fats that have not been heated in the course of cooking or food processing above the temperature of boiling water. If unsaturated fats are overheated by themselves they produce a series of mutagenic products. However when fat is overheated in cooking it is usually associated with meat or fish or eggs or other food rich in protein. The fat is either an inherent part of the food or is added as in frying.

MUTAGENS PRODUCED BY COOKING AT HIGH TEMPERATURES

Highly mutagenic substances are produced by heating protein and these mutagens appear to be responsible for most of the mutagenicity of the average
diet. A study of the Dutch diet, supported by both Dutch and American govern-
ment agencies found that much of the mutagenicity of the average Dutch diet
was caused by cooking (Alink *et al.*, 1988). Food was prepared with a composition matching average Dutch food consumption. A first set of pellets was
made from raw components before cooking and had only a low mutagenicity,
indeed had no detectable mutagenicity in the first test. The same raw food
'after processing under usual household conditions (at approximately 150°C)'
was clearly mutagenic in the Ames test used in this study. Addition of fruit
and vegetables reduced but did not eliminate the mutagenicity of the cooked
food pellets. Three of the mutagens responsible for the mutagenicity were
identified and were found to be the same as previously identified in fried beef
by other research workers. This Dutch study had many obvious limitations.
Many antimutagens apparently act by energizing digestive enzymes and a mix-
ture of foods in laboratory tests would not for this reason alone be expected
to show the same mutagenicity as in the digestive tract. The choice of 150°C
as an average cooking temperature in Dutch kitchens may be correct but mutagen production increases rapidly above this temperature which is often exceeded both in the home and in commercial cooking.

As part of a study at the University of California seven 'fast food' restaur-
ants offering grilled hamburgers were visited and it was reported (Bjeldanes
et al., 1982):

> 'Of the seven restaurants we sampled two provided hamburgers with consistently high
> mutagen content, three with consistently low mutagen content, and two showed consid-
> erable variation between sampling times. Precise data on the cooking times and tempera-
> tures of the hamburgers are not available. However, discussion with each vendor indicated
> a qualitative correlation of higher mutagen content with more severe cooking conditions,
> including the use of increased temperature associated with the sporadic high values oc-
> curring when the cook was rushed.'

The hamburgers in this study varied in mutagenicity by a factor of over 50
in the Ames test. The mutagenicity of beef, pork or eggs increases as the
cooking temperature increases from 150°C to 300°C and they become charred.
Mutagenicity increases with cooking time as well as temperature and may
vary by a factor of 100 or more. The Dutch experiments excluded mutagens
produced at these higher temperatures. It has been shown that mutagens are
produced in beef and beef extract by boiling at 100°C (Commoner, 1978).
However the mutagens at 100°C are negligible compared with those produced
at the higher temperatures. Boiling or braising protein around 100°C does not
make a serious contribution to the mutagenicity of any diet.

The digestive tract provides a first line of defence against the ingress of
mutagens. If the contents of the human digestive tract were always antimut-

agenic doubts about the desirability of overheating protein might be unjustified. Many mutagens are wholly or partly destroyed during digestion. Small samples of people from Canada, Japan, South Africa, USA and elsewhere show that some people have antimutagenic faeces and that for them any absorption of mutagens from the digestive tract is presumably very small. However there are people who have mutagenic, even highly mutagenic, faeces, and mutagens may then be absorbed. The first line of defence against mutagens can be breached. Baker *et al.* (1982) showed that about one-third of the potent mutagenic activity in fried bacon and pork reappeared in the urine of human subjects very quickly after they were eaten. The increase in the mutagenicity of the urine by a factor of 10 or more persisted for about 12 hours and then declined to normal in another 12 hours. The meat was not charred but fried in its own fat at temperatures of 150–190°C. Sjödin and Jägerstad (1984) reported that fried meat mutagens fed to rats are partly absorbed and that the urine then becomes mutagenic. Hayatsu *et al.* (1985) showed that mutagens from fried meat eaten by humans made their urine mutagenic. Hayatsu commented:

'Our results on the effect of beef ingestion are consistent with the pork and bacon results in terms of the acute nature of the response. The present study has demonstrated that this phenomenon can take place under normal, everyday eating conditions'.

Accordingly Hayatsu examined the mutagenicity of urine of volunteers after their everyday meals. Figure 6.7 shows for one man the mutagenicity of urine lingering after a fried beef lunch and 6.8 for the same man after a fried beef dinner. Lindeskog *et al.* (1988) of the Karolinska Institute, Stockholm, has shown experimentally in rats that if fried meat is consumed every day the mutagenicity of faeces particularly, but also of urine, is cumulative and increases for at least a week with a diurnal cycle. Mutagens from fried meat are carried by the blood to all body systems and are possible mutagenic agents

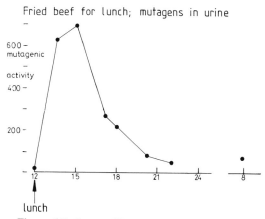

Figure 6.7. Source: Hayatsu *et al.*, 1985, Figure 2.

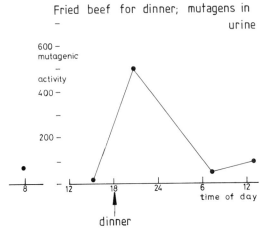

Figure 6.8. Source: Hayatsu *et al.*, 1985, Figure 3.

for the germ line. One of the beef protein pyrolysis products has been shown to be a potent mutagen in hamster ovary cells (Thompson *et al.*, 1987).

Sugimura and Nagao of the National Cancer Center, Toyko, as long ago as 1982 said that it was not yet possible to decide on the comparative importance of different mutagens but nevertheless:

'Based on recent information it seems wise to reduce exposure to these mutagens as much as possible. This would probably be possible without disturbing the quality of life. For instance, it would be simple to avoid charring food.'

Three years later Sugimura said there was 'no doubt about the necessity' of reducing the formation and consumption of mutagens in cooked food (Sugimura, 1985).

REDUCING THE MUTAGENICITY WITHIN THE DIGESTIVE TRACT

Dion *et al.* (1982) of the Ludwig Institute of Cancer Research, Toronto, has shown the effect on faecal mutagenicity of a dietary supplement of 400mg of both vitamin C and vitamin E daily. Vitamin C and E are both antioxidants. These vitamins may not be such effective antimutagens as chlorophyll or have such a wide spectrum but they have both been shown to inhibit the formation of the mutagenic nitroso compounds or to destroy them (Newmark & Mergens, 1981; Bruce *et al.*, 1979; Newberne & Suphakarn, 1983). The variation from day-to-day in the faecal mutagenicity of a single donor on a controlled diet or on a controlled diet with a supplement of vitamins C and E is shown in Figure 6.9. It is seen that the faecal mutagenicity declined steadily from the first of the 15 days when the vitamins were taken and the decline was particularly rapid during the first 3 days. There was a 3 week interval between the taking of the controlled diet without the two vitamin supplements and the

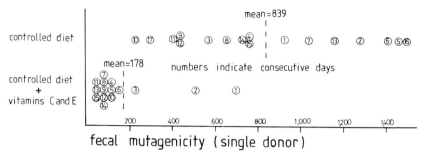

fecal mutagenicity (single donor)

Figure 6.9. Reduction of mutagenicity within digestive tract by vitamins C and E on consecutive days. Source: Dion *et al.*, 1982, Figure 1.

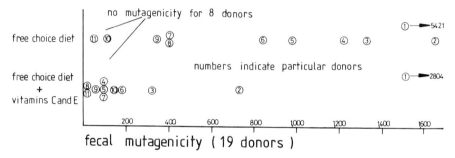

fecal mutagenicity (19 donors)

Figure 6.10. Reduction of mutagenicity within digestive tract by vitamins C and E in 11 donors. Source: Dion *et al.*, 1982, Figure 2.

15 days that included supplements. Examination of faeces does, of course, show only the end result of the conflict between mutagens and antimutagens higher up the digestive tract. Figure 6.9 suggests that vitamins C and E have the capacity to reduce digestive tract mutagenicity in some cases. The effect of vitamins C and E on the digestive tract mutagenicity of 19 donors is compared in Figure 6.10. It is seen that there were 8 donors with no measurable mutagenicity. Faeces as already noted can be antimutagenic so that the contents of the donors' digestive tracts may in these cases have had little effect, or even a negative effect, on their mutation rate. However, 11 of the 19 students had faeces that were mutagenic in different degrees and faecal mutagenicity was reduced by factors up to 10 or 15 by the supplements of vitamin C and E for 15 days. The antimutagenic effect of the vitamins lasted about 3 weeks but then declined. The great variability of faecal mutagenicity between the 19 donors is apparent as well as the variability from day to day seen in Figure 6.9. Donor number (1) in Figure 6.10 is seen to have had a mutagenicity of higher order than the remaining 18 and although the vitamin supplements reduced the faecal mutagenicity of donor number (1) they did not reduce it to the level of the other donors.

The impression from the study by Dion is that 9 or 10 out of the 19 students would have benefited from a higher habitual consumption of vitamin C and

E. Recommended daily intakes of these vitamins cannot be soundly based only on systemic requirements after absorption. These nutrients are needed and partly used up, as are also the unsaturated fatty acids, within the digestive tract where most of the mutagens in a normal diet are destroyed. These two vitamins also destroy some of the mutagens produced during digestion.

The effects of dietary fibre on the mutagenicity of faeces and urine were studied by Lindeskog *et al.* (1988). The mutagens used were from fried meat; again boiled meat was found not to be mutagenic. The results showed no effect of the fibre on the mutagenicity of urine. The effect on faecal mutagenicity varied widely between types of fibre. Pure cellulose had no useful effect but other fibres reduced faecal mutagenicity and the Swedish study concluded:

'The clearest effects were seen with wheat bran where a considerable part of the total mutagenicity was bound to the fibre pellet at the pH values prevailing in the gastro-intestinal tract. For the other fibres the results were less clear.'

Canadian research on faecal mutagenicity has also reported that a diet containing whole grains rather than refined cereals produces lower mutagenicity (Kuhnlein *et al.*, 1981, 1983). The same studies report that diets containing 'relatively high levels of fruits, vegetables and dietary fibre' produce a relatively low faecal mutagenicity. These studies also showed that by change of diet it was possible to reduce faecal mutagenicity from a high to a low level in a fortnight. The dietary fibre that is effective appears to be that contained in whole grains or vegetables. The studies on faecal mutagenicity emphasize the importance of vegetables, fruit and whole grains in limiting the mutagenicity of the digestive tract. They also emphasize the difficulty of neutralizing the mutagens produced by overheating meat.

So far naturally occurring mutagens in food have not been discussed, because there is very little published evidence that in the diets of the developed world they have any influence on mutation rates. The flavanoids are, for example, a family of chemicals that occurs naturally in many plants and some widely distributed members are mutagenic while others are antimutagenic. However the same fruits and vegetables generally contain antimutagens. Black currants contain flavanoids but also have an exceptionally high content of antimutagens. The mutagens are presumably destroyed at an early stage of digestion. In Japan a list of vegetables has been published which Japanese housewives have been advised to eliminate from their kitchens, but none of these are familiar in Europe (Sugimura and Nagao, 1982). The young shoots of bracken (*Pteridium aquilinum*) have been regarded as a delicacy in Japan and many other countries, but are certainly mutagenic and carcinogenic and are perhaps a reminder that everything that tastes agreeable is not necessarily safe (Stavric *et al.*, 1984). The greatest danger from these naturally occurring mutagens may be that they can become separated from their associated antimutagens in cooking or processing, which may destroy the antimutagens while some more stable mutagens remain. Such naturally occurring mutagens may also be more dangerous to individuals with an already enhanced mutagenicity of the contents of the digestive tract.

The cells of the lining of the digestive tract are among those that replicate most frequently among all the cells of the body throughout life. It might therefore be expected that chronic exposure of the lining of the digestive tract to mutagenic contents could cause or aggravate digestive disorders by interfering with the renewal of the lining. The association of ulcerative colitis, Crohn's disease and coeliac disease with raised mutation rates has been reported and is discussed further in Chapter Eight (Emerit *et al.*, 1972, 1979; Konstantinova & Bratanova, 1969).

SOME CONCLUSIONS

The present chapter has discussed mutagens and antimutagens in diet and in the digestive tract. In conclusion it may be said that it is not apparent that food need necessarily result in a mutagenic content of any part of the digestive tract or make any positive contribution to the human mutation rate. However it often does.

What is then the course of wisdom for couples planning a pregnancy? The period of greatest susceptibility to most mutagens is around conception and it is therefore at this time that antimutagens are most important. All, or nearly all, fresh vegetables and fruit ordinarily on sale contain antimutagens and lower mutation rates and there are no substitutes. The prospects of manufacturing compounds that are equally effective, or of recovering the compounds from plants are limited. Some of the naturally occurring antimutagens have high molecular weights and are chemically unstable and heat sensitive. The antimutagenicity of fresh vegetables and fruits depends upon a range of compounds each with its limited antimutagenic spectrum. The value of many reasonably stable antimutagens like the catechins is in doubt and awaits evaluation. The task of evaluating even one naturally occurring antimutagen for human preventive purposes is formidable. The first practical conclusion follows: Young men and women of reproductive age should aim to have a low mutation rate and are therefore well advised to eat ample fresh vegetables and fruit. There are many studies based on epidemiological and other evidence about heart disease, cancer and other disorders which also arrive at the conclusion that an ample consumption of fresh vegetables and fruit is wise at all ages (US National Research Council, 1982; Armstrong *et al.*, 1975; Wynn & Wynn, 1979).

A second practical conclusion relates to cooking. The latest research suggests that most of the mutagens in the average diet are not contained in the raw food but are produced by pyrolysis of protein, and these mutagens are not all destroyed in the digestive tract but some are absorbed and penetrate all body systems. These mutagens are not produced at the temperature of boiling water or of braising, but by grilling, roasting or cooking at high temperatures in fats and oils. Young men and women who are planning pregnancy are advised to limit the occasions when they eat meat, fish, eggs, cheese or other protein food that has been cooked at temperatures much above those of boiling water. The pathological consequences of pyrolysis products entering the body via the lungs is no longer doubted; tobacco smoke is a familiar hazard. There is no reason for supposing that the potent pyrolysis products that enter the body from the digestive tract are not also harmful at all ages. Urine can be made mutagenic by pyrolysed protein in food as well as by inhaling the smoke from pyrolysed tobacco.

Protection of the human genome requires a low mutation rate during the susceptible periods around the time of conception. A low mutation rate requires both avoidance of exposure to the products of pyrolysis and an antimutagenic diet.

7. Infectious illness before conception

THE CASE FOR AVOIDING CONCEPTION DURING INFECTIOUS ILLNESS

That herpes virus can cause visible damage to chromosomes was first reported in *Nature* by Hampar and Ellison in 1961. Since that time many other viruses have been shown to be mutagenic and it was suggested in *Mutation Research* in 1986 that all viruses are mutagenic and that they are a significant cause of inherited congenital defects in man (Gershenson, 1986). Some other microorganisms including the rickettsiae and mycoplasmas, that spend part of their life cycle within cells, are another ubiquitous cause of mutation (Halkka & Halkka, 1969; Kundsin *et al.*, 1971). In populations in which the adults lack immunity to viral diseases such as measles, mumps and chicken pox they have dramatic effects on reproduction. For example measles and influenza epidemics on Pacific islands have been reported to reduce birth-rate by 80 per cent 9 months after the epidemic (Smith, 1960). Numbers of men and women still reach reproductive years without immunity to chicken pox, measles, mumps and whooping cough in the United Kingdom in spite of immunisation of children. These childhood fevers can cause congenital malformation and stillbirth (Hurley, 1983). Figure 7.1 shows the rise and fall in mutation rates as indicated by chromosomal breaks in cultured leucocytes following the onset of infection (Aula, 1965).

The damage done to the male germ cells of mice by influenza virus in the laboratory is illustrated in Figure 7.2. Most early miscarriages are a consequence of mutations of parental germ cells, as shown in Chapter Two from the study of early abortuses. Aneuploidy is the commonest type of mutation associated with early miscarriage, which is perhaps the commonest outcome of a mutation before and around conception. It would therefore be expected that viral diseases which are mutagenic would cause miscarriage. The literature of centuries states that this is indeed so. Finland (1973) quoted Hippocrates' first treatise on 'Epidemic Diseases' describing the effects of influenza: 'All my acquaintances miscarried that chanced to be with child'. The long history of influenza is marked by great differences in the apparent potency of the virus and in the susceptibility of populations and individuals. Miscarriage was reported in 25 to 40 per cent of pregnancies during the 1918 influenza pandemic in the USA and the case-fatality rate of pregnant women averaged about 10 per cent (Harris, 1919). In contrast the Asian influenza epidemic in the autumn of 1957 caused very few casualties among pregnant women, but a study at the Johns Hopkins Hospital, Baltimore, showed that among serologically confirmed cases of influenza during the first trimester of pregnancy there

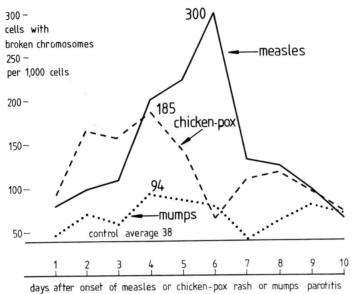

Figure 7.1. Mutagenicity of some viral diseases in human cells.
Source: Aula, 1965, Figure 3.

Mutagenicity of influenza virus

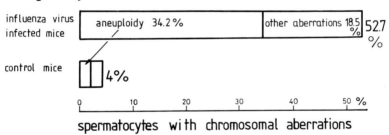

Figure 7.2. Source: Sharma & Polasa, 1978, Tables 1 to 4.

was a significant increase in casualties notably of miscarriages and births with congenital malformations (Hardy *et al.*, 1961).

The history of most diseases shows great contrast between their impact on different populations. In one report from Saudi Arabia 35 per cent of pregnancies complicated by hepatitis ended in miscarriage or stillbirth and there was a high mortality among the pregnant women (Gelpi, 1970). Well-fed pregnant women in Munich apparently infected by the same hepatitis virus had no increase in miscarriage, low birthweight or perinatal mortality compared with controls who were not infected (Dorfler & Voigt, 1966).

Figure 7.3 shows the raised mutation rate caused for a few days by chicken pox as indicated by chromosomal breaks in lymphocytes. It is seen in this

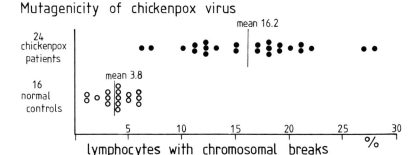

Figure 7.3. Source: Aula, 1965, Figure 2.

diagram that uninfected normal controls had an average 3.8 per cent of lymphocytes with chromosomal breaks. Micronuclei are chromosomal fragments and their number provides another measure of DNA damage. The numbers of micronuclei per 1,000 lymphocytes in 45 healthy people aged 20 to 40 years are shown in Figure 7.4. The random distribution among 45 hypothetical people is shown for comparison, assuming a constant probability of occurrence of micronuclei of 9 per 1,000 lymphocytes. The comparison shows that the variations in micronuclei numbers among the real people were not random, with constant probability, and were not therefore caused by some constant influence.

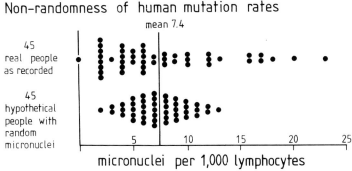

Figure 7.4. The non-random variability of micronuclei between "healthy" donors aged 20 to 40. Source: Fenech & Morley, 1985, Figure 4.

Eight of the samples from real people had only 2 micronuclei and one sample had 23 micronuclei, results that could not have happened by chance if the 45 real people were, like the hypothetical people, equally at risk. There are major variations in mutation rate between people. A very high mutation rate is characteristic of serious illness and micronuclei per 1,000 lymphocytes can exceed 500. When easier and cheaper methods have been developed for estimating mutation rate it is likely to be used more widely as an indicator of illness. Mutation rate is a useful concept used widely in the literature, but has severe limitations with present methods of measurement. Thus the mutagenicity of the blood fluctuates from day to day and even between evening and morning. It is not generally known how old micronuclei or chromosomal abnormalities in somatic cells are, but it is assumed or implied in many studies that they had their origins in the recent past.

Most of the many causes of mutation in man and animals have been studied using somatic cells, for example leucocytes. Techniques have now been developed for studying the chromosomal abnormalities of human sperm directly; Brandriff *et al.* (1985) at the University of California investigated the chromosomal integrity of 2,468 sperm cells from 11 donors. Figure 7.5 shows the spread in the apparent mutation rates in the sperm cells of the 11 men from 1.9 to 15.8 per cent, with an average of 7.7 per cent. Most of the aberrations were chromosomal breaks, but the frequency of aneuploidy ranged from 0.6 to 3.1 per cent. Blood samples were available for 10 of the donors and investigation of lymphocytes showed that 9 out of 10 had a higher frequency of chromosomal aberrations in their sperm cells than in their lymphocytes. The substantial variation in mutation rates between individuals is seen to be as apparent in the mutations in germ cells as in blood cells. Viral diseases may not be responsible for the large variations in mutation rate of apparently normal individuals. There are many other causes of mutation. There is nevertheless little doubt that some germ cell mutations are caused by viruses and that it is wise to postpone conception while either parent is suffering from a viral infection and for long enough afterwards for damaged germ cells to be eliminated.

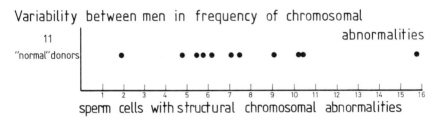

Figure 7.5. The non-random variability of chromosomal abnormalities in sperm cells between "normal" donors. Source: Brandriff *et al.*, 1985, Table 1.

Not all viral diseases are serious or life-threatening but it is important for couples to understand that benign everyday viral diseases cause temporary increases in mutation rate. Upper respiratory infections are the commonest illnesses reported to family doctors and the common cold has been reported to increase mutation rates (Kurvink *et al.*, 1978). Infections such as tonsilitis have been reported to reduce sperm count and motility temporarily, reflecting a slow-down in DNA synthesis without the sufferers being seriously ill (David, 1982). Secondary infections by bacteria have not been shown to increase mutation rates.

In times of even mild, benign illness there is an increased consumption of a variety of drugs both off-prescription and prescribed. Watanabe (1979) of the Niigata University School of Medicine studied the embryonic chromosomal anomalies associated with the taking of drugs during the three weeks before and three weeks after the first day of the last menstruation. Data were obtained by karyotyping abortuses obtained by elective abortion. Results are summarized in Figure 7.6 which shows for all drugs, and for all analgesics and antipyretics, a significant increase in chromosomal anomalies associated with drug taking. The number of embryos with chromosomal anomalies (26/117) was too small to show statistical significance for individual drugs separately. A later paper from the same school emphasized that most of the chromosomal anomalies were associated with illness notably acute respiratory illness as well as with the medication (Yamamoto *et al.*, 1982). It can only be said that either or both the illness and medication may have caused the chromosomal anomalies. There are other studies showing that under some circumstances aspirin is mutagenic to sperm (Meisner & Inhorn, 1972).

Is it then possible to find out which drugs are mutagenic in what Watanabe calls the perifertilization period? Good information is only available for a very few drugs in spite of an efficient information retrieval service for mutagens and teratogens (EMIC-UK). The literature discourages the use of any drugs by women and by men during the susceptible periods around conception. One review refers to the majority of drugs selected from different pharmacologic classes as spermicidal (Peterson & Freund, 1975). Another study of 10 antibiotics in rats and one in man found that they interfered with the multiplication of spermatogonia or interfered with meiosis I if the spermatocytes survived to this stage. The paper concluded: 'This action of antibiotics seems specific to germ cells' (Timmermans, 1974). As spermatogonia are affected a period of 4 months may be needed to eliminate damaged sperm and recover fertility after a course of antibiotics.

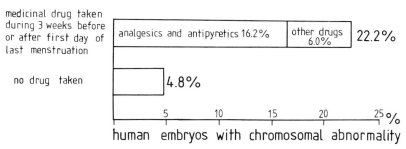

Figure 7.6. Mutagenicity of medicinal drugs taken around conception.
Source: Watanabe, 1979, Tables VI and X. Reprinted by
permission of S. Karger AG, Basel.

THE CASE FOR AVOIDING INFECTIONS IN ANTICIPATION OF CONCEPTION

Twenty years ago a treatise on prenatal illness concluded a chapter on viral embryopathy by recommending that women should become immune as far as possible to such diseases as rubella, measles, mumps and poliomyelitis before reaching maturity, and that during the preconception period and the first trimester of pregnancy women should where possible avoid exposure to infection (Thalhammer, 1967). In the United Kingdom rubella is still thought to be responsible for 2 to 3 per cent of congenital mental retardation (Ho-Yen & Joss, 1988). It may be desirable to check the titre of rubella antibodies as part of preconception care (Chamberlain & Lumley, 1986).

The long history of listeriosis illustrates the vigilance necessary to avoid foods infected with organisms damaging to reproduction. A Swiss monograph on listeriosis was published in the early 1960s (Seeliger, 1961). Thalhammer (1967) referred to listeriosis as the infection most serious in some communities in its consequences to reproduction. Lang (1955) showed that in rural communities as much as a third of children in the age range 1 to 15 years with brain damage had at some stage, and probably in utero, been exposed to listeriosis. Unpasteurised milk and cheese made from unpasteurised milk are major sources of listeriosis. Inadequate refrigeration can seriously increase the risk.

Infection with the parasite *Toxoplasma gondii* is thought to be responsible for 2 to 3 per cent of congenital mental retardation. Under-cooked meat is a major source of toxoplasmosis. Cat faeces and therefore litter trays are another source. The current recommendations for avoiding undercooked meat and unclean cats should be extended from pregnancy to the prepregnancy period. Toxoplasmosis can also cause miscarriage.

Cytomegalovirus (CMV) is reported to be the cause of some 10 per cent of congenital mental retardation in the UK (Hurley, 1983). Infection with CMV is generally asymptomatic in women and there is no specific vaccine or other treatment. Infection can be readily diagnosed from blood samples but tests are unlikely to be done in the absence of symptoms. Infection by CMV is however, like infections with other herpes viruses, a disease of opportunity. Low birthweight infants growth-retarded in utero have increased susceptibility to many infections and to the herpes viruses in particular (Templeton, 1970). CMV infection can be chronic but probably only in a host with a defective immune status. A diet before conception that reduces the risk of intrauterine growth retardation will also reduce the risk of embryonic and foetal infection and damage to germ cells (Chandra, 1988).

Sexually transmitted diseases (STDs) are an important group that affects pregnancy outcome and reduces fertility. A consensus report on STDs of the US Institutes of Health concluded that there were 2.5 million cases in the USA each year of nongonococcal urethritis and related chlamydial infections (Wiesner & Parra, 1982). There has been a shift in prevalence from the larger organisms of syphilis and gonorrhoea which are comparatively easy to diagnose, and are amenable to effective antibiotics, to much smaller organisms which are more difficult both to diagnose and to treat, such as chlamydia and the mycoplasmas, papilloma and herpes viruses and HIV viruses. A scholarly book of 652 pages published as recently as 1973 entitled, *Obstetric and Perinatal Infections*, did not mention chlamydia or papilloma or HIV viruses (Charles & Finland, 1973).

The risk of infection from casual sexual contacts has increased but is very unpredictable. There are reports of more than 10 per cent of women in some populations within the developed world being infected with chlamydia and higher percentages with one or other type of STD. The infected women who became pregnant were at greater risk of what was described in a symposium on chlamydial infections as 'the constellation of abortion, prematurity, stillbirths and neonatal death' (Thompson *et al.*, 1982).

STDs are a major cause of infertility. Population Reports from Johns Hopkins published a review in 1983 of infertility and sexually transmitted disease and concluded:

'For both men and women, the most common preventable cause of infertility is infection... Pelvic inflammatory disease in women, due to sexually transmitted disease (STD) and other infections, probably accounts for more than half of all female infertility in many regions. Although the woman is usually blamed when a couple cannot have children, male factors explain about one-third of all infertility. Low sperm count, often the result of infection, is the most important male factor.'

The major percentage of women found to be infertile by the number of episodes of pelvic inflammatory disease (PID) is shown in Figure 7.7 based on a study by Weström (1980). PID is often difficult to treat as it may become

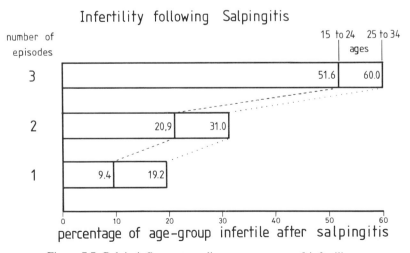

Figure 7.7. Pelvic inflammatory disease as a cause of infertility.
Source: Weström, 1980, Table IV.

a focus of multiple opportunistic infections. Weström and Mårdh (1983) of the University Hospital, Lund, concluded a review in the British Medical Bulletin:

> '...Now and for many years to come we will have to harvest the seed of the STD and salpingitic epidemic of the 1960s and 1970s in terms of the many women deprived of the possibility of motherhood because of postinfection tubal damage'.

Throughout much of the world the epidemic has continued since the 1970s.

The 1981 consensus report of the US National Institutes of Health concluded that one of the commonest STDs to prejudice male fertility is chlamydia (Wiesner & Parra, 1982):

> '*Chlamydia trachomatis* is the major cause of nongonococcal urethritis (NGU) in men, which is twice as common as gonorrhoea. Chlamydia causes more than one-half of the 500,000 cases of epididymitis occurring each year. This painful complication of NGU is potentially sterilizing.'

In the United Kingdom chlamydia is reported to be the commonest sexually transmitted pathogen, causing 35 to 40 per cent of cases of so-called 'nonspecific' infection (Alexander, 1988). Fifteen to 17 per cent of chlamydia is reported in asymptomatic patients attending clinics.

Population Reports (1983) suggests that as many as 20 to 25 per cent of nongonococcal urethritis cases in the USA are caused by mycoplasmas. Mycoplasmas, like the chlamydial organisms, can ride on spermatozoa and reduce motility (Chang *et al.*, 1984; Wolner-Hanssen & Mårdh, 1984). The evidence that mycoplasma infection reduces male fertility is more convincing than its effect on the female (Toth *et al.*, 1980). The mutagenicity of mycoplasmas was, however, reported by Kundsin *et al.* in 1971 and has been confirmed in many subsequent studies. The full human consequences of mycoplasma infection remain to be explored. These organisms adhere to sperm, enter the uterine cavity and the fallopian tubes causing obstruction.

Genital herpes is an STD associated with miscarriage, low birthweight, malformations and foetal infection (Hurley, 1983) and is mutagenic as shown in Figure 7.8 from Ghosh and Ghosh (1983) in cell culture experiments using blood lymphocytes from infected patients and controls. The frequency of sister-chromatid exchange used in this study is an indicator of chromosomal damage. Genital herpes is generally regarded as a localized infection confined to the genitalia but Ghosh and Ghosh showed that genital herpes multiplies in the genitalia and is released into the blood and that the amount of chromosomal damage is linearly related to the amount of antibody in the case of both types of herpes. The resulting viraemia affecting all body systems may be very slight in a patient with a healthy immune system. Herpes is, however, a fatal disease among ill-fed peoples in the developing world.

The papilloma viruses, named after the warts or papillomas that they cause, are another family of STDs, with a reported incidence in England & Wales

Mutagenicity of herpes

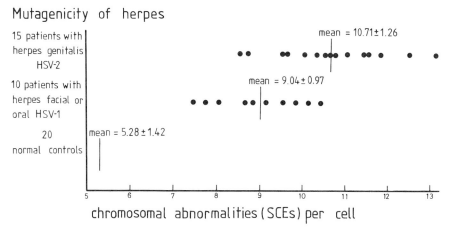

Figure 7.8. Mutations in somatic cells of herpes patients.
Source: Ghosh & Ghosh, 1983, Table 1.

higher than for herpes virus. The prevalence of papilloma virus in the USA and Europe has been increasing (Blank, 1986). Papilloma viruses like herpes viruses are more serious in immunosuppressed or ill-fed people. Papilloma viruses are also mutagenic and cause chromosomal aberrations in the cells that they infect (Evered & Clark, 1986).

The increased prevalence of some STDs is partly a consequence of the increased mobility of people. The number of persons travelling between cities and between countries has increased and is forecast to continue to increase. No doubt the prevalence of syphilis and gonorrhoea would have increased if it were not for the excellent medical services, armed with antibiotics for treatment, available in the United Kingdom and elsewhere. Syphilis and gonorrhoea are not reported to be mutagenic. The viral diseases are a more difficult and increasingly serious problem. Papilloma and herpes viruses and indeed chlamydia are already the subject of a substantial literature suggesting that they cause cancer and in particular cervical cancer responsible for about 2,000 deaths of women every year in the UK. Unlike chemicals or radiation viruses can produce mutations at specific locations in somatic and germ cells which are peculiar to the particular virus types. Many of the consequences of STD viral infection have yet to be discovered. The current publicity about HIV infections and AIDS has shown to the public the great difficulty in treating virus diseases. A leading article about HIV in the British Medical Journal concluded (9 August 1986):

'True, the virus has been isolated; but so have the viruses of hepatitis, influenza, rabies, and other fatal diseases, and we still have no treatments. All the evidence suggests that the development of a vaccine will prove immensely difficult.'

For generation after generation it has been the men and women sensitive to dangers to themselves and their families who survived. Wise men and women will adapt to a more dangerous sexual environment. The concept of survival has a special meaning for men and women who choose to live together and wish for children. For them survival means successful breeding of the next generation. Survival requires protection of their own health and reproductive capacity. During preconception consultations the doctor can convince a couple that casual sexual contacts are not consistent with their aim of survival with this extended meaning. It is not only that the rheumatic pains of Reiter's syndrome for the man, or the miseries of PID for the woman, are not compatible with a satisfactory life, but to risk an STD is to risk not only an important part of your own life purposes but those of your present or future partner and children on which your happiness will depend as much as upon your own health.

8. Premature ageing in men and women can affect reproduction

In the 1950s Penrose of University College, London (1955), studied the ages of the parents of babies with birth defects believed to have been caused by gene mutations. He concluded:

> 'The influence of the father's age is shown to be of critical significance. When the effect of the father's age on incidence is appreciable, as in achondroplasia, the hypothesis of fresh gene mutation as the cause is strengthened.'

Achondroplasia is the commonest form of skeletal dysplasia leading to dwarfism. An organization was formed in 1960 called, The Little People of America, open to individuals under 58 inches (147cm) in height. A team at Johns Hopkins University co-operated with the LPA to compile information of value in counselling achondroplastics and their parents (Murdock *et al.*, 1970). In a series of 148 cases it was found that 31 achondroplastics had one or both parents affected, but in 117 cases there was no family history of achondroplasia. Father's age at the birth of the child was available in 102 cases and has been used in Figure 8.1 where an exponential curve has been fitted to the data. The risk of achondroplasia increases exponentially with the age of the father.

The prevalence of many other diseases increases with age and the increase generally follows curves that are approximately exponential over the age range used in Figure 8.1. Age-specific mortality rates from many causes also increase exponentially with age. Indeed the age-specific mortality for all diseases shown for the USA in Figure 8.2 is approximately exponential at the lower ages. Figure 8.1 relates, however, only to a small minority. Figure 8.2 relates to a minority of individuals who as a result of illness aged prematurely. It is everyday experience that some people age more rapidly than others and this is apparent from the mortality curves from most causes of death. Figure 8.1 describes a male mutation rate that increases with age producing a condition in offspring, achondroplasia, but as it relates only to a small minority of fathers it prompts the question: Do all men have a mutation rate that increases exponentially with age or only a minority? Figure 8.2 then also prompts further questions: Are there particular diseases that accelerate ageing and also increase mutation rate thus affecting reproduction? Ageing is inevitable, but premature ageing may not be inevitable and disorders responsible for premature ageing

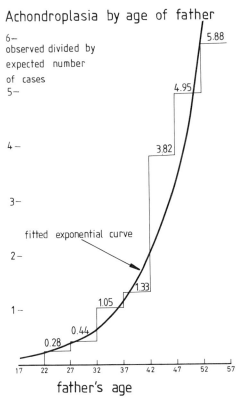

Achondroplasia by age of father

Figure 8.1. The increase in male mutation rate with age.
Source: Murdoch *et al.*, 1970, Table 4.

may be prevented, or treated to delay their effects. Are the mutations in male germ cells leading to congenital disorders an inevitable and inescapable result of ageing, or can the risk of mutations be reduced in some cases by treatment of illnesses associated with premature ageing?

Achondroplasia is an example of a disorder caused by an autosomal dominant mutation with a frequency estimated to vary from 15 to 100 cases per million births in different countries. Each particular, specific autosomal dominant mutation is rare but 1,443 (+1,144 not fully validated) types are described in McKusick's catalogue (1988). Vogel (1984) shows graphically the increase of mutation rate for some of these diseases with paternal age. The number of such distinct dominant mutations described in the literature continues to increase. Friedman (1981) estimated that the risk of a father aged over 40 having offspring with autosomal dominant disease was between 0.3 and 0.5 per cent and that this was about one-third of all babies with diseases due to new autosomal dominant mutations.

The age of a man at the conception of his children may affect the health of his grandchildren. Thus a mutation in a father's X-chromosome carried by

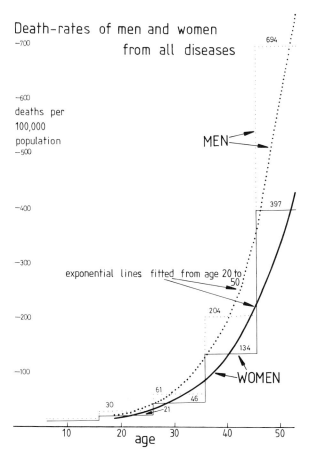

Figure 8.2. Age-specific death-rates of men and women from all causes, USA 1978.
Source: World Health Organisation, 1981.

his daughter may not be expressed in the daughter but only in his grand-son. McKusick (1988) lists 139 (+171 not fully validated) X-linked diseases. Haemophilia A is such an X-linked disease and is shown in Figure 8.3 to increase in prevalence with the age of the sufferer's maternal grandfather at his mother's conception (Herrmann, 1966). The rate of increase with age of these grandfathers is very similar to that for the age of the father in achondroplasia and an exponential curve fits the data well. Duchenne muscular dystrophy is another X-linked disorder. X-linked diseases can also be produced by maternal mutations but are commoner in the male. One paper from the University of Colorado says (Lubs, 1981):

'The results from this study suggest that the mutation rate in the haemophilia gene in sperm cells is two to four-fold greater in sperm than in egg cells.'

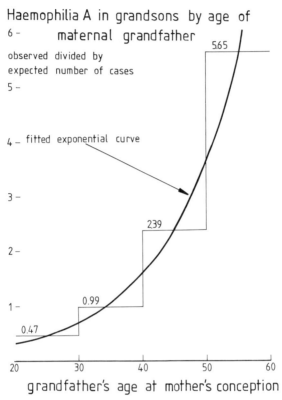

Figure 8.3. The risk of X-linked disease increases with age of grandfather.
Source: Herrmann, 1966, Figure 1.

Karp (1980) in the American Journal of Medical Genetics commented on the
increased mutation rate with age:

> 'Such a high rate of gene mutation due to advanced paternal age would have considerable
> implications for genetic counselling. For example, should we be encouraging obstetricians
> to screen for 'pregnant husbands' over the age of 40 and offer them counselling, as they
> would do for women over 35?'

This writer concluded that the 'primary educational thrust' should be aimed
at the non-pregnant, prepregnant population to encourage child-bearing before
age 35:

> 'Some of them might plan differently if they knew that there existed a risk of undiag-
> nosable, serious genetic disease due to advanced paternal age. It seems to make sense
> in terms of the overall prevention of birth defects to advise men as well as women to
> have their children, if possible, before the age of 35 or 40. Such an approach would
> probably benefit not only the immediate offspring, but subsequent generations as well.'

This general advice to parents is repeated in other medical journals (Jones *et al.*, 1975; Stoll *et al.*, 1982). This advice is not, however, appropriate for all men or the majority of men if the increase in risk with age is a consequence of the premature ageing of a minority. The advice is also not useful to parents already in their late 30s or to their medical advisers. The question that may perhaps be useful is whether the prospective father belongs to the minority with an exceptionally high mutation rate and if so whether treatment is possible. This question can only be useful for prospective fathers and it is too late when wives are already pregnant.

DISEASES WHICH CAUSE PREMATURE AGEING

Mutation rate varies more between individuals from causes unconnected with age than it does by increase in age during the reproductive years. An increase in the average number of chromosomal anomalies with age has been shown in somatic cells (Schneider, 1978, 1980). An increase in the average number of micronuclei or chromosomal fragments in lymphocytes with age has also been found (Fenech & Morley, 1985). However these studies show great variations between individuals. Some men in their 20s have more micronuclei than other men in their 60s and 70s. Furthermore the number of micronuclei only about doubled between the ages of 30 and 60 in Fenech and Morley's investigations and the 'increase in mutation rate with donor's age' was attributable to a minority with high rates. It has also been shown in *in vitro* experiments that the proliferative capacity of human cells declined with the age of the donor, but that the cells of some donors in their 60s and 70s had a greater proliferative capacity than other donors in their 20s and 30s (Martin *et al.*, 1970). Doubt is also thrown on these and other experiments by their choice of 'healthy' individuals as donors because by doing so they were excluding most of the individuals with high mutation rates and with rates increasing most rapidly with age. The evidence suggests that much if not all the increase in rates with age is attributable to individuals who are not healthy or are manifestly ill.

The ageing of germ cells might be thought of as proceeding throughout adult life at a rate which is independent of other body systems. The evidence suggests on the contrary, as discussed in earlier chapters, that the integrity of germ cells depends throughout life upon the hormonal and nutrient content of the blood and furthermore that germ cells can be seriously damaged and mutated by viruses at any age. It is therefore to be expected that the ageing of germ cells is associated with the ageing of other body systems. A disease affecting a particular body system begins the premature ageing associated with chronic disease and an increased mutation rate. The increased human mutation rate associated for example with multiple sclerosis is illustrated in Figure 8.4 (Emerit & Marteau, 1971; Unglaub-Leisten *et al.*, 1975). The raised mutation

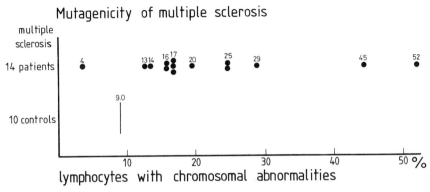

Figure 8.4. Source: Emerit & Marteau, 1971, Table 2.

Mutagenicity of ulcerative colitis and Crohn's disease

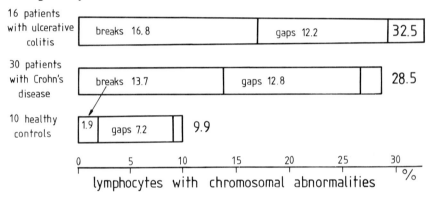

Figure 8.5. Source: Emerit *et al.*, 1979, Table 1.

rates associated with ulcerative colitis and Crohn's disease are illustrated in Figure 8.5 (Emerit *et al.*, 1972, 1974). Rheumatoid arthritis and a variety of other rheumatic diseases have been reported to be associated with raised mutation rates (Sherer *et al.*, 1981). There is a variety of uncommon inherited diseases for example Fanconi's anaemia which are associated with chromosomal instability and raised mutation rate (Schroeder-Kurth *et al.* 1989). These particular diseases have in common that they are associated with microscopic lesions leading to sclerosis. The repair of all tissues, and wound-healing, requires DNA and RNA synthesis and the raised mutation rate is evidence of a reduced rate of DNA synthesis and repair. Emerit *et al.* (1974) found that the blood serum from patients with scleroderma is mutagenic in the culture of cells from normal individuals. An aberration in the composition of blood serum, resulting from a disease which produces a raised mutation rate, may damage germ cells before conception and may continue to disturb reproduction after conception.

Diabetes is one of the ageing diseases that increases mutation rate in men. Fairburn *et al.* (1982) from the University of Oxford summarized 7 studies which showed that between 35 and 59 per cent of male diabetics were impotent. Sexual disturbances were found in men with only mild metabolic disturbance who were leading a normal life. Diabetic men have depressed hormonal responses, as illustrated in Figure 8.6 for the gonadotrophin responses to LH-RH in male diabetics (Distiller, 1975). The reduced androgen levels result in reduced spermatogenesis and in particular in a reduced rate of replication of spermatogonia. Diabetes has been listed as one of the disorders responsible for premature ageing (Goldstein, 1978). Ando *et al.* (1984) from the University of Calabria and Ghent reported depressed levels of the androgens testosterone and dehydroepiandrosterone in diabetics and concluded:

'Diabetes could have a similar effect to that of ageing suggesting a precocious alteration in both gonadal and adrenal secretion in male diabetics.'

Both the incidence of diabetes and the mortality increase approximately exponentially with age like the incidence of autosomal dominant diseases with father's age. United States returns for all races show an incidence in 1982–5 of 5.8 per 1,000 for males under 45 rising to 52.6 per 1,000 in the age range 45 to 64. Male mortality from diabetes in the USA is shown in Figure 8.7 to increase approximately exponentially with age up to about age 50.

Diabetes is only one example of an endocrine disorder that affects the outcome of pregnancy. A survey was conducted of 2,779 individuals in Whick-

Depression of pituitary response in diabetic men

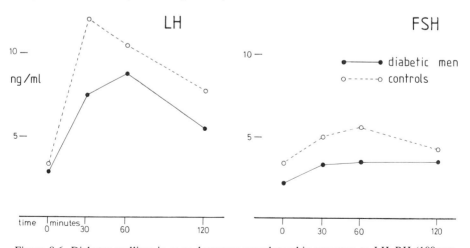

Figure 8.6. Diabetes mellitus in men depresses gonadotrophin response to LH–RH (100mcg injected at time zero). Source: Distiller *et al.*, 1975, Figure 1. Reprinted by permission of the American Diabetes Association.

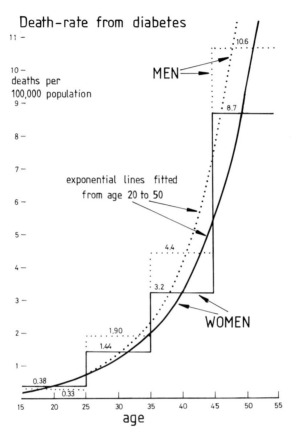

Figure 8.7. Age-specific death rates of men and women from diabetes, USA 1978. Source: World Health Organisation, 1981.

TABLE 8.1

COMPARATIVE PREVALENCE OF DIABETES AND OF THYROID DISOR-
DERS IN MEN AND WOMEN, COUNTY DURHAM, 1977, 2,779 PEOPLE.

	percentages		
	female		male
overt hyperthyroidism	1.9–2.7		0.16–0.23
overt hypothyroidism	1.4–1.9		0.10
subclinical hypothyroidism	7.5		2.8
overt diabetes		0.8	
high fasting glucose level		1.8	

Source: Tunbridge *et al.*, 1977.

ham, County Durham to determine the prevalence of thyroid disorders (Tunbridge *et al.*, 1977). Table 8.1 compares the prevalence of thyroid disorders and diabetes. This study suggests that thyroid disease may be comparable in prevalence to diabetes. Bakke *et al.* (1975) at the University of Washington showed that partial removal or impairment of the thyroid in male animals before mating to a normal female produces birth defects in the offspring. Some of these defects, when compatible with survival, were found to be heritable. Thyroid disease, like diabetes, is mutagenic in male as well as female. However the levels of both clinical and sub-clinical disorder at which male mutation rate is seriously increased is not well enough established to estimate the comparative importance of diabetes and thyroid disorders. In cases of overt hyperthyroidism drug treatment is usual and effective. The drugs given, such as propylthiouracil, if given in excess do, however, produce hypothyroidism and therefore can be mutagenic if dose is not very well controlled.

Thyroid disorders, diabetes, multiple sclerosis, ulcerative colitis, rheumatoid arthritis, pernicious anaemia are associated with raised mutation rates. These are diseases that have an increasing prevalence with age and are responsible for at least an important part of premature ageing. The fathers who are ageing prematurely can identify themselves or be identified and can be helped. There are treatments for most of the ageing diseases that can at least reduce risks.

An increase in mutation rate with age cannot be explained by any increased exposure to radiation or smoke or pyrolysed protein or mutagenic chemicals. A simple linear accumulation of mutations with age would not produce the exponential curves associated with the risk of mutagenic disease from the ageing of fathers or mothers. The exponential curve is the most basic of all curves generated by circular processes. Diabetes mellitus is one example of a mutagenic disease that affects not only germ cells but is thought to be caused partly by somatic mutation, in this case within the immune system, causing autoimmune disease within the pancreas (Adams *et al.*, 1984). Mutation is part of the process of premature ageing. The conclusion of the studies briefly reviewed here is that chronic diseases in men should receive attention in anticipation of a pregnancy equal to that advocated presently for a woman.

THE PREMATURE AGEING OF WOMEN CAN AFFECT CHILDBEARING

An association between diabetes and birth defects has been the subject of reports for more than a century. Lecorché (1885) wrote many years before the advent of insulin:

'If diabetes does not always completely prevent fertilization, it seems to cause profound impairment of the products of conception, subverts nutrition, shortens life or causes developmental defects incompatible with life.'

Diabetes in women is prominent among the diseases of premature ageing that affect reproduction (Kram & Schneider, 1978). In the USA the reported incidence of diabetes in women in 1979–81 was 6.9 cases per 1,000 women under age 45 rising to 55.1 cases for women aged 45 to 64 (US National Center for Health Statistics, 1987). The steep increase in incidence with age is reflected in the exponential increase in mortality with age of women from diabetes shown in Figure 8.7.

Diabetes is an endocrine disorder and might be expected to disturb gonadotropin secretion in women as in men. Diabetes does in fact depress the hypothalamic-ovarian axis as illustrated in Figure 8.8 showing a depressed response to 100 µg of LH-RH by 22 diabetic women (Distiller *et al.*, 1975). All except two were on insulin therapy, but were tested before the morning dose which was delayed. The depression of gonadotrophin levels prompts many questions about the effects of diabetes on reproduction. Is the premature increase of womens' infertility with age partly a consequence of diabetes? How far does diabetes increase the risk of birth defects? Is diabetes partly responsible for the increased risk of chromosomal abnormalities including Down's syndrome with maternal age? Is diabetes mutagenic? A Leader in the Lancet said (22 March 1980):

'If preimplantation, and perhaps even preconceptual, stages of development are vulnerable to the effects of maternal diabetes then clearly the management of diabetes needs to precede conception.'

Depression of pituitary response in diabetic women

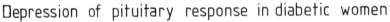

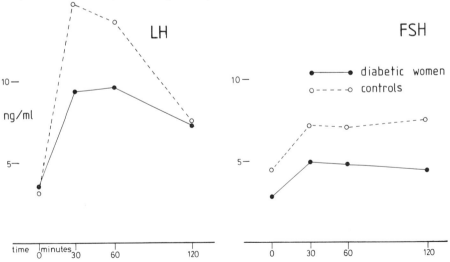

Figure 8.8. Diabetes mellitus in women depresses gonadotrophin response to LH–RH (100mcg injected at time zero). Source: Distiller *et al.*, 1975, Figure 1.
Reprinted by permission of the American Diabetes Association.

Chromosomal anomalies in embryos of diabetic mice

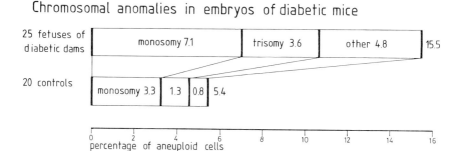

Figure 8.9. Mutagenicity of diabetes in mice. Source: Endo and Ingalls, 1968, Tables 2, 3, 4.

This quotation poses the question as to whether diabetes does affect female germ cells.

Japanese-American teams at Niigata and Boston Universities were the first to report that diabetes is mutagenic in female mice and interferes with meiosis causing diverse chromosomal abnormalities (Endo & Ingalls, 1968). Diabetes in female mice was found to be associated with chromosomal breakage, polyploidy and aneuploidy in the cells of embryos removed 19 days after mating. The percentages of the cells with aneuploidy are shown in Figure 8.9. The mice were made diabetic with alloxan and were mated within two weeks of treatment. Ninety-eight per cent of the control mice were fertile but only 44 out of 200, or 22 per cent of the treated mice. Twenty per cent of the diabetic mice had one or more malformed foetuses including 13 with serious malformations, for example cranioschisis, spina bifida, hernia and cleft palate. Two malformed foetuses had over 90 per cent of abnormal chromosomes. The alloxan intake was adjusted so that it did not cause infertility on the one hand and was not too low on the other hand to produce any effect (Endo, 1966). The diabetes produced casualities only at critical levels of severity and caused infertility if more severe. In a later Japanese study of diabetes in mice, also using alloxan, ova were harvested only 3½ days after mating at about the 16-cell stage. The aneuploidy, the polyploidy and chromosomal gaps and breaks were found to be present already at this stage (Yamamoto *et al.*, 1971). The authors stress that ovulation was disturbed and most chromosomal anomalies probably had their origin before mating.

The effects of diabetes on ovulation in female rats have been studied without using diabetogenic drugs at the Institute of Physiology in Buenos Aires by Chieri *et al.* (1969) who removed part of the pancreas. Diabetes reduced the rate at which ova matured within the ovary before ovulation and also reduced the number of ova ovulated. The ovulation rate in these experiments was quickly restored by insulin. Furthermore insulin restored ovulation rates more quickly than it restored blood glucose to a normal level. The authors of this study concluded:

> 'Insulin therapy was able to restore the number of eggs to a normal level suggesting that the ovulatory disturbance was related critically to the insulin deficit.'

Ovulation in these animal experiments was unaffected by high or low blood glucose levels if the insulin levels were normal. It was the insulin levels that were found to be critical during ovulatory maturation and conception. In the culture of cells in the laboratory insulin is also a critical and essential component of the culture medium for most types of cell including human cells.

Because diabetes depresses the hypothalamic-gonadal axis in both men and women it would be expected to cause infertility. Before the discovery of insulin from 95 to 98 per cent of diabetic women were reported to be infertile (Gellis & Hsia, 1959). Insulin is highly effective in restoring fertility. It is, however, much easier to restore fertility than to ensure a satisfactory birth outcome.

Diabetic management has reduced the perinatal death rate impressively in recent years, but there have been many reports of increases in malformation rates among survivors. Ballard *et al.* (1984) discussed this history and listed a number of studies up until 1980 reporting malformation rates ranging up to 20 per cent with a typical figure around 10 per cent for the children of diabetic mothers. Ballard reported a major malformation rate of 16.8 per cent for the years 1970–78 from the University of Cincinnati for diabetic pregnancies that had only been managed after diagnosis of pregnancy. Diabetic management needs to precede conception to prevent birth defects.

AGE-DEPENDENT AND AGE-INDEPENDENT AETIOLOGY

There are many causes of raised mutation rate such as influenza, or a temporary nutritional deficiency, or exposure to a mutagenic chemical which are unrelated to parental age. An inherited propensity such as a translocation is also unconnected with parental age. It would therefore be expected that some part of the prevalence of birth defects would be independent of age and another part would be a function of age. Writers on ageing over many years have used models to represent morbidity and mortality which included one term to represent the age-independent component and a second term for the age-dependent component, generally exponential. Greenwood (1928), an actuary, suggested that the age-dependent term represented 'physiological constitution' in contrast to the age-independent term reflecting enviromental causes, for example transport accidents. Lamson & Hook (1980) applied this model to Down's syndrome and Table 8.2 shows in 5 populations the proportion of cases that are apparently independent of maternal age and those which are age-dependent. Figure 8.10 is a diagrammatic representation separating the numbers of cases of Down's syndrome that would have been expected at the

TABLE 8.2

PROPORTION OF CASES OF DOWN'S SYNDROME ATTRIBUTABLE TO
CAUSES DEPENDENT AND INDEPENDENT OF MATERNAL AGE: SUM-
MARY OF 5 STUDIES.

Population	independent of age	dependent upon age
	percentages	
Massachusetts	36.3	63.7
Sweden	50.7	49.3
New York	40.4	59.6
Australia	45.3	54.7
British Columbia	45.8	54.2

Source: Lamson & Hook, 1980.

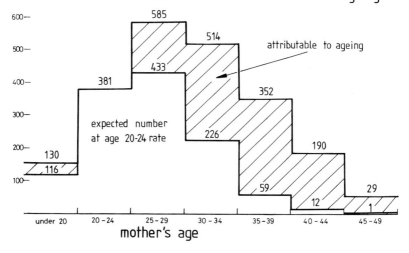

Figure 8.10. Partition of Down's incidence into age-dependent and age-independent causa-
tion. Source: OPCS, 1983.

rate for age 20 to 24 and the numbers attributable to the ageing effect; 54 per
cent in this figure were age-independent and 46 per cent age-dependent. Friedman (1981) superimposed the frequency curves of Down's syndrome and
maternal age, and achondroplasia and paternal age and showed that they were
very similar.

The prevalence of every type of birth defect can be roughly divided for
any particular population into parental age-independent and age-dependent
components. The age-dependent components are substantial for Down's syndrome and for most other birth defects associated with chromosomal abnormalities. Figure 8.11 shows the increased incidence of Down's syndrome

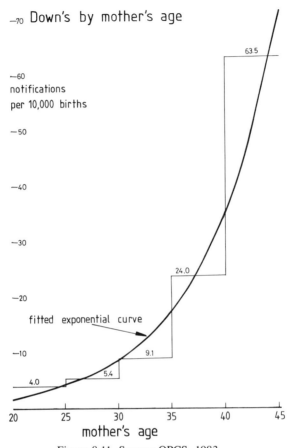

Figure 8.11. Source: OPCS, 1983.

notifications with maternal age, and Figure 8.12 the notifications of other chromosomal abnormalities with maternal age, both figures using data for England and Wales. The risk of most birth defects increases with maternal age but for most types, for example for congenital heart disease, the age-dependent component is much smaller than for birth defects associated with chromosomal abnormalities.

Diabetes is a prominent disease of premature ageing and would be expected to be particularly associated with the birth defects including chromosomal abnormalities with their large maternal age-dependent components of risk. Down's, Klinefelter's and Turner's syndromes are the three commonest one-generation genetic diseases associated with chromosomal abnormalities. An association between diabetes and these three genetic diseases would be expected from the animal experiments described above which showed that critical levels of diabetes produced chromosomal abnormalities including trisomy and by the evidence that depression of the hypothalamic-gonadal axis can

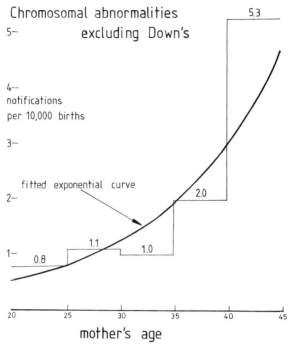

Figure 8.12. Source: OPCS, 1983.

cause non-disjunction, and that diabetes is one of many disturbances that causes such depression (Hansmann, 1984).

There are studies from several countries showing an association of parental diabetes and the three major syndromes associated with chromosomal abnormality. Navarrete *et al.* (1967) reported from the First Obstetric Hospital, Mexico City, abnormal glucose tolerance tests of 9 out of 12 mothers of Down's syndrome babies. Milunsky (1969) of Tufts' University, having found a family history of diabetes in 209 out of 393 children with Down's syndrome, made a detailed study of the parents of 42 Down's syndrome children and found that 16 (38 per cent) showed abnormality in a glucose tolerance test compared with 6.8 per cent of 176 controls with normal children. Forbes and Engel (1963) of Harvard Medical School reported an association between diabetes and chromosomal anomalies in female babies. They studied 41 cases of Turner's syndrome and related disorders characterized by developmental failure of the female gonads. The patients all had defective or absent ovaries associated with the absence of one X chromosome or a defect in this chromosome, the results of a new mutation in one parent. In 20 out of 41 patients there was a family history of diabetes and in 14 the diabetes was on the father's side only. The incidence of diabetes in the families of the 41 patients was 10 times higher than in the general population of Oxford, Massachussetts.

Three years later it was reported from Denmark, Italy, Argentina and the USA that diabetic parents were overrepresented among the parents of male babies suffering from Klinefelter's syndrome, another one-generation genetic disease characterized by male infertility and generally an extra X chromosome resulting from non-disjunction at meiosis I or II. The results of the four studies are aggregated in Table 8.3. It is seen that almost a quarter of the Klinefelter children had a diabetic parent and that 12 out of 23 diabetic parents were fathers. Again the incidence of diabetes in both mothers and fathers of the Klinefelter children was significantly higher than would be expected for any normal population with at most 1 or 2 per cent of diabetics among people in the childbearing ages.

The Leader in the Lancet (22 March 1980) referred to the 'desirability of fastidious diabetic control' when planning a conception. The prevention of birth defects, including chromosomal aberrations, requires more careful control of diabetes before and around the time of conception than does the restoration of fertility or reduction of perinatal mortality. Preconception care of diabetics is a matter for a specialist hospital clinic and many such clinics are now providing such care. However primary care has the difficult initial responsibility for referring patients to specialist clinics for diagnosis and management. There is much evidence that in every country the coverage of such clinics is limited. Some women reporting to a diabetic clinic for the first time have suffered from diabetes for some years. Some women only reach a diabetic clinic too late when already pregnant. Other diabetic women are never referred to a diabetic clinic at all by the primary care services but refer themselves.

One of the first prepregnancy clinics for diabetes was established in 1976 at the Royal Infirmary in Edinburgh (Steel *et al.*, 1982). Clear accounts of the experience of the Edinburgh clinic emphasize the care and persistence needed by both patients and clinic staff to achieve the tight control of blood compo-

TABLE 8.3

DIABETES MELLITUS IN PARENTS OF PATIENTS WITH KLINEFELTER'S SYNDROME; SUMMARY OF 4 STUDIES

country		number of patients	with diabetes		percentage of patients with diabetic parent
			fathers	mothers	
Argentine	a	32	4	3	21.8
Denmark	b	31	2	6	25.8
Italy	c	8	3	1	50.0
U.S.A.	d	24	3	1	16.7
total		95	12	11	24.2

Sources: a Wais & Salvati, 1966; b Nielsen, 1966; c Menzinger *et al.*, 1966; d Zuppinger *et al.*, 1967.

sition needed. The results of such intensive diabetic control reported by Fuhrmann from the Institute for Diabetes, Karlsberg, are summarized in Figure 8.13 with a larger sample of women. Hospitalisation for a limited period before conception to achieve optimum control and to teach self-management was shown to be effective (Fuhrmann *et al.*, 1983).

By combining the results of numbers of small studies from different countries as separated as Argentina, Denmark, Italy, and the USA, as in Table 8.3 for Klinefelter's syndrome, and from Mexico and the USA for Down's syndrome and Turner's syndrome it may be concluded that about 20 per cent of these disorders might be prevented by strict preconception control of diabetes. The data on which this conclusion is based is manifestly unsatisfactory. The cost of Down's syndrome alone in every country is formidable and would justify the collection of adequate data throwing light on its etiology.

The US Collaborative Perinatal Studies covered 23,000 white women of whom 1.8 per cent had 'overt diabetes' and were on 'insulin or analog therapy'; and 17.7 per cent of these 424 women had babies with major malformations (Chung & Myrionthopoulos, 1975). This study showed an increase by a factor of 3.5 in the risk of CNS malformations to 24 per 1,000 births. Zacharias *et al.* (1984) have reported 19.5 cases per 1,000 of babies with neural tube defects born to white diabetic mothers and 18.0 per 1,000 to black diabetic mothers, increases in both cases more than 10 times that of the non-diabetic births of 1.4 and 0.8 per 1,000. Diabetes increases the risk of many other types of congenital malformation. In no country are the data that have been found good enough to estimate the percentage of total birth defects associated with diabetes of either father or mother. Assuming that 1.6 per cent of women who become pregnant have a degree of insulin deficiency enough to increase the risk of malformations by a factor of 5, then this deficiency would be responsible for 8 per cent of all malformations. The available data are such that this can be no more than a tentative hypothesis. The actual figure could be higher, but it is apparent that men and women who are not diabetic have most of the children

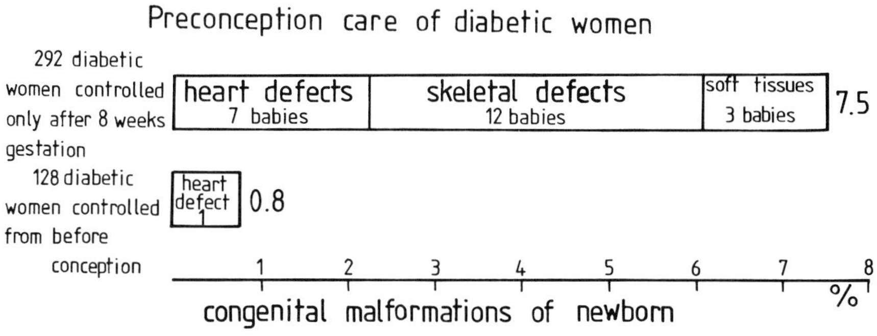

Preconception care of diabetic women

Figure 8.13. Efficacy of diabetic control before conception. Source: Fuhrmann, 1983, Table 2. Reprinted by permission of the American Diabetes Association.

with malformations and that diabetes cannot even be the only age-dependent disorder concerned.

Diabetes is a slowly progressive autoimmune disease in which the cells of the immune system, notably the T-cells, slowly destroy the islet cells of the pancreas that produce insulin (Powers & Eisenbarth, 1985). Diabetes is only one autoimmune disease and others include hypothyroidism, Graves' disease, multiple sclerosis, pernicious anaemia, arthritis. The prevalence of these disorders overlaps with diabetes and some 10 to 12 per cent of women diabetics have been reported to develop thyroid disease and 2 or 3 per cent to develop pernicious anaemia (Beral *et al.*, 1984). Another report shows 23 per cent of 144 diabetic women as developing arthritis of autoimmune origin (Cruickshanks *et al.*, 1984). The autoimmune origin of diabetes prompts the question as to whether there is any evidence of an association between the birth of children with chromosomal abnormalities and other autoimmune diseases.

Hypothyroidism is among the autoimmune diseases overlapping with diabetes. Case histories of an association of Down's syndrome and hypothyroidism go back to Stölzner (1919). Myers (1938) in Canada found 9 times the prevalence of thyroid disease among the mothers of Down's syndrome children compared with controls. Benda (1949), writing about Down's syndrome, said:

'Thyroid anomalies are so frequently seen that they are an important link in the chain of events. The common denominator is a threshold of sterility.'

Thyroid (T_3) deficiency like insulin deficiency slows down ovulatory maturation causing infertility, and there is a grey area between infertility and normal ovulation in which meiosis I can be slowed down producing chromosomal abnormalities. Ek (1959) examined 41 mothers of Down's children and found that the thyroid gland was pathologically enlarged in 12, but none had any severe physical disease; the frequency of goitre in the same part of Sweden was 1.1 per cent. The mothers of the 41 Down's children had an average protein bound iodine (PBI) significantly higher than normal. Fialkow *et al.* (1971) reported 17 per cent of 177 mothers of children with Down's syndrome as having clinical thyroid disease compared with 6 per cent of controls, who were mothers of children with a variety of disorders mainly mental retardation but who were not known to carry chromosomal abnormalities. Thirty-four per cent of the mothers of Down's syndrome children had abnormal levels of thyroid antibodies compared with 15 per cent of controls. Nielsen (1972b) listed 5 different studies with a total of 348 mothers of Down's syndrome children of whom 30.7 per cent had increased thyroid antibodies compared with 13.8 per cent of controls. There is an association between Down's syndrome and maternal thyroid deficiency. Thyroid disease is mutagenic in animals as already noted (Bakke *et al.*, 1975). Partial thyroidectomy in female rats before mating produces a range of congenital malformations (Langman & Faassen, 1955). Thyroid hormone (T_3) is essential like insulin in cell culture.

The Whickham survey concludes (Tunbridge *et al.*, 1977):

'There is clearly a large reservoir of autoimmune thyroid disease in the community and clinically obvious hyperthyroidism and hypothyroidism are only the extreme ends of the spectrum.'

The percentage of women with raised thyrotrophin (TSH) levels increased with age from 4.0 per cent under age 25 to 17.4 per cent over 75, the increase being steepest between 35 and 55, and 12.3 per cent of women had palpable and visible goitres.

Both thyroid disease and diabetes point to autoimmune disease in general as one important cause of chromosomal abnormalities. It cannot however be assumed that the hormonal deficiencies associated with these diseases act directly on germ cells. They depress the hypothalamic-gonadal axis and this alone can disturb meiosis and produce a range of chromosomal abnormalities. There are many papers that discuss the origins of autoimmune disease from which it may be concluded that the part of the genome concerned with the immune system is particularly susceptible to damage by mutagenic influences. As most if not all autoimmune diseases increase mutation rate they are self-generating but could also be initiated by viruses or other mutagens. There are reported cases of viral diseases, for example congenital rubella, causing diabetes and viruses can induce diabetes experimentally in mice. Viruses are, however, only one cause of mutation.

9. Conclusions

THE IMPORTANCE OF THE PROSPECTIVE FATHER

1. The time is ripe for greater attention to fathers' contribution to the outcome of pregnancy. The contribution of fathers varies in a complicated way from one population to the next according to cultural traditions, endemic disease and differences in the habits of men and women. A growing understanding of fathers' role has been one of the changes of the last 30 years. The US Collaborative Perinatal Study 1958–65 of 55,908 women and their pregnancies collected no information on fathers except their incomes. The British Perinatal Mortality Survey 1958 collected no information on fathers except their occupation or social class when available. In response to the growing awareness of the dangers of smoking the German prospective, multi-centre Perinatal Study, 1964–70, included information in the design about fathers' smoking as well as mothers' (Koller, 1983). Details of smoking by fathers were available for 6,714 out of 7,870 pregnancies and about 46 per cent of fathers smoked regularly. This German Study showed that smoking by the father when the mother did not smoke was associated with an increased rate of early and late miscarriage, preterm birth, low birthweight, perinatal death and the occurrence of severe congenital malformations. Figure 9.1 shows from this study a statistically significant association of higher perinatal mortality and fathers smoking. Figure 9.2 shows the association of all severe congenital malformations with father smoking regularly. For every mother who smoked there were 4.2 fathers who smoked and fathers contributed correspondingly more smoking-

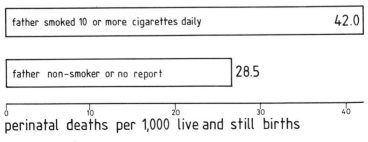

Figure 9.1. German multi-centre survey of risk factors in pregnancy:
12 obstetric and 15 paediatric hospitals; 7,870 single births 1964–70.
Source: Koller, 1983, Table 4.3.9–12.

Severe congenital malformations by fathers' smoking

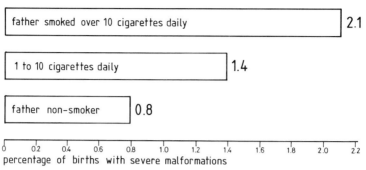

Figure 9.2. German multi-centre survey of risk factors in pregnancy:
Source: Mau & Netter, 1974, Table 8.
Reprinted by permission of Georg Thieme Verlag, Stuttgart.

linked malformations. This study suggests that fathers share responsibility with mothers for miscarriage, perinatal death and congenital malformations. Damage to fathers' germ cells, or mutations, are responsible for some part of such unfavourable outcome of pregnancy.

2. Women hoping to have a family at any time should be helped to stop smoking before that time comes. The well-recognized danger of women smoking in pregnancy extends to the prepregnancy period (US Surgeon-General, 1980).

ONE-GENERATION GENETIC DISEASE RESULTING FROM MUTATION IN A PARENT

3. It should be more widely understood that the risk of many one-generation genetic diseases, and indeed diseases inherited by grandchildren, can be reduced by avoiding causes of mutation. These genetic diseases include Down's syndrome and other chromosomal disorders, autosomal dominant disorders like achondroplasia, X-linked disorders like haemophilia, a part of epilepsy, schizophrenia and mental subnormality. Research has continually added to the list of disorders known to be caused in whole or in part by new mutations in germ cells and embryonic cells. This knowledge has increased in step with the increasing understanding of the importance of new mutation in somatic cells in the aetiology of cancer. Research on mutation was motivated from its beginning by concern to protect the human genome and genetic heritage. It only became apparent gradually as research proceeded that much human disease was a consequence of damage to the genome within somatic and germ cells in the not so distant past.

4. Concern should not be limited to protection from mutagens that cause specific, easily identifiable disease but should extend to protection against anything which, like tobacco smoke, increases human mutation rate. Mary Lyon said in *Nature* in an article entitled: 'Measuring mutation in man' (Lyon, 1985):

> 'Major advances in preventing the birth of genetically affected children are being made, through genetic counselling, prenatal diagnosis and the use of recombinant DNA methods. But mutation remains a problem, resulting in the levels of many genetic diseases being maintained despite adverse selection, and it is becoming increasingly important to assess the possible increase in mutation rates caused by chemical or physical agents in the environment... If the mutation rate rises the incidence of such mutationally maintained diseases will rise, so efforts are being directed towards the detection of mutagens in the environment and their control or elimination.'

Mary Lyon then refers to the work of the International Commission for the Protection against Environmental Mutagens and Carcinogens (ICPEMC). There are many chemicals in the environment not yet assessed for mutagenicity.

THE GROWING LIST OF CAUSES OF MUTATION

5. That not only radiation but chemical compounds can cause mutations has been known since the 1930s and 40s (Auerbach & Robson, 1946). Intake of mutagenic xenobiotics is one of the causes of raised human mutation rates. It was in the 1960s that governments world-wide became more concerned about chemical damage to the human genome and the environmental mutagen societies were formed in many countries. The journal *Mutation Research* was established in 1964 and one of the early British contributions was about chemically induced mutations in mice (Cattanach, 1966a, 1966b, 1982). The dominant lethal test for mutagenicity using treated male animals and unexposed females was described in 1972 (Epstein & Röhrborn, 1970; Epstein *et al.*, 1972), and has been adopted world-wide (Burger *et al.*, 1989). This test depends upon the capacity of mutagens to cause damage to male sperm. At least 30 chemicals which are mutagenic have been found in tobacco smoke and go far to explain the effects on pregnancy outcome of smoking by fathers and mothers.
6. When prescribing drugs which are known to be mutagenic or which may be mutagenic the possible intention of the patient to start a pregnancy should be considered. There are, of course, circumstances when the prescription of a mutagenic drug, for example morphine, or the use of X-rays are in the best interests of the patients. Couples should confide their intentions, and should when possible postpone conception following the use of mutagenic drugs or X-rays.
7. When possible men and women planning a pregnancy should avoid self-treatment with off-prescription drugs. Drugs reported, often belatedly, to be

mutagenic are freely available and sold in substantial quantities in many countries without any weighing of costs and benefits by consumer or supplier. An example is paracetamol reported to be mutagenic in animals and in man (Hongslo *et al.*, 1988; Kocisova *et al.*, 1988). Analgesics have been suggested as an important cause of miscarriage (Watanabe, 1979).

8. Ideally alcohol should not be consumed by men and women hoping to conceive. Alcohol consumption increases the risk of miscarriage (Harlap & Shiono, 1980; Kline *et al.*, 1980). Alcohol affects all levels of the hypothalamic-gonadal axis and can depress levels of gonadotrophins (Gavaler & Van Thiel, 1987). Animal experiments have shown that alcohol interferes with meiosis I and II and can cause chromosomal abnormalities including non-disjunction (Badr & Badr, 1975; Kaufman, 1985). Alcohol consumption is particularly ill-advised around the time of meiosis I and II in men and women (Cicero, 1982). A whole number of Mutation Research in 1987 (volume 183 No. 3) was devoted to papers of the International Commission on the genotoxicity of alcohol (Bridges, 1987).

9. It is wise for men and women to avoid unnecessary consumption of food containing xenobiotic food additives throughout the susceptible periods surrounding conception. Some substances are so widely used as hardly to be thought of as additives. Thus, for example, Arnold & Boyes (1989) have reviewed over 200 papers and the results of over 200 tests on the mutagenicity of saccharin, some negative and some positive. A part of the mutagenicity of commercial saccharin manufactured in Europe, America, Japan, Korea and China has been caused by impurities. It has also been reported that bacteria in the digestive tract cause saccharin to react with amino acids to produce new mutagenic products (Lawrie *et al.*, 1985). The published studies on the mutagenicity, teratogenicity and carcinogenicity of saccharin now cover more than 20 years and show no sign of coming to a conclusion, illustrating the high cost of testing a chemical for mutagenicity when its market is already established and the mutagenicity is challenged. Saccharin is at most a mild mutagen but the mildness may well be offset for the individual who uses saccharin several times a day. About 75 per cent of saccharin production is used in soft drinks and one can may contain 150mg. In 1976 about 3 million kilograms of saccharin were consumed in the USA.

AVOIDING HUMAN CASUALTIES BY USE OF ANIMAL STUDIES

10. Disaster races to meet those who wait for proof of danger. The results of bacterial and animal tests should be respected as there is no other way of avoiding human casualties. DES (diethylstilboestrol) is a drug now known to be mutagenic (Banduhn & Obe, 1985). DES was reported to be carcinogenic in animals in Germany and the USA (Pierson, 1936; Shimkin & Grady, 1940). It was, however, only in 1971 that it was first reported that maternal DES

therapy was associated with vaginal adenocarcinoma of their daughters. Claims for damages in the Courts have exceeded $1 billion. This was described in the US Congress as 'trial by catastrophe'.

11. The Environmental Mutagen Information Centre (EMIC), United Kingdom Office, which operates a computer retrieval service for all mutagens and teratogens should be more widely used (EMIC-UK). This service is linked to Oak Ridge National Laboratory in the USA. The historical record shows that many casualties caused by mutagenic chemicals and drugs can be attributed to failure to heed published information including the results of animal studies.

12. When no medical cause of miscarriage, or infertility or birth defect can be found chemical mutagens in the work place can be suspected and may be found to be known mutagens. DBCP (dibromo-chloropropane) is a pesticide widely used at one time particularly in California and provides a cautionary tale. DBCP was reported to cause atrophy and degeneration of the testes of rats, guinea pigs and rabbits by Torkelson *et al.* (1961). DBCP is mutagenic. Sixteen years passed before the first of a long series of papers was published on the impairment of reproductive function, particularly of male workers, engaged in the production or use of DBCP.

13. A prospective father or mother who suspects there may be dangers at work should consult the safety representative of their Trade Union, the personnel department or the medical staff. There are many drugs and chemicals on which EMIC cannot yet provide adequate information. Employees are also sometimes exposed to mixtures of unknown composition. Safety limits for some mutagens are published but observance of these limits requires measurement in the workplace which is not always done. Furthermore the safety limits which may be acceptable to prevent toxic signs or symptoms in the adult, may not be strict enough to prevent damage to germ cells. The United Kingdom Regulations relating to exposure of employees to lead are, for example, much less strict than the corresponding United States regulations which purport to protect both 'males or females who wish to plan pregnancy' (US Department of Labor, 1978). Dangers from some of the commoner chemicals used in industry are discussed by Barlow & Sullivan (1982) and by Fletcher (1985).

THE TEMPORARY DEFERMENT OF CONCEPTION

14. Spacing of births by at least 2 years is wise. Many risks to the following baby increase as the spacing falls below 2 years. At least 15 months from the birth of one child before risking the next conception is a wise rule for couples.

15. A temporary or passing illness of a woman or her partner is a good reason for postponing a conception for 3 or 4 months. Mutation rate is increased by infectious illness especially by viral disease, and therefore by such temporary, transient illnesses as influenza and the common cold. Men and women at the

time of a conception should try to have been fit and well for a length of time that includes the period of heightened susceptibility of their germ cells. Drugs taken at the time of such temporary illness may also increase mutation rate.

16. Women and their partners with any sign or symptom of chronic illness should confide in their family doctor and should be advised to postpone conception until they have seen a consultant physician. Most of the casualties that might have been avoided by specialist care today, but are not avoided, are the consequence of men and women being referred too late. Thus most of the congenital malformations of children born to diabetic parents can be prevented if the parent or parents are referred to a clinic for careful management of the diabetes well before conception. The same is true of other disorders such as hypothyroidism and some types of anaemia. There is substantial evidence of underdiagnosis of both diabetes and hypothyroidism early enough before conception.

17. Thin women should postpone conception until body weight has been corrected. The 165 women in the Hackney study who had babies in the optimum birthweight range had a mean BMI of $23.7kg/m^2$ (Doyle *et al.*, 1990a). The average BMI is around $24kg/m^2$. The risk of low birthweight, congenital malformation and other handicapping conditions increases as the BMI falls below $24kg/m^2$ and American data show 50 per cent of women infertile below $20.7kg/m^2$ (Frisch, 1977). Experiments in animal husbandry have shown that it is best for fertility and outcome for animals to conceive on a rising and not a falling body weight (Morrow, 1980a, 1980b).

18. A leaflet for women entitled, *Getting Fit for Pregnancy* implies that it is wise to postpone a conception until fitness is achieved, and a second, *Thinking about a baby? A man's guide to preconception health*, implies that a man's health may also be grounds for postponement (Maternity Alliance, 1990). Many family doctors in the British National Health Service give preconception advice or have their own preconception clinics. In Britain there is a series of some 50 clinics in private medicine offering preconception care (Foresight, 1990). A book summarising the advice of these clinics recommends a six month period of improvement in health for men and women in preparation for a conception (Barnes & Bradley, 1990). Such preparation is the most constructive part of family planning and must require postponement of conception, but for widely differing lengths of time.

THE MODULATION OF MUTAGENICITY BY NUTRITION

19. A diet adequate in calcium, magnesium, iron and zinc protects against the heavy metals lead and cadmium. Animal experiments suggest that lead may be the most important mutagen in the contemporary human environment, affecting pregnancy outcome at blood concentrations not infrequently encountered among the less well fed (Wynn & Wynn, 1982).

20. Poor nutrition increases susceptibility in different degrees to most if not all mutagens and teratogens and thereby increases mutation rates. Thus well fed rats, for example, tolerate thalidomide (Giroud *et al.*, 1962). However deficiencies of riboflavin, pantothenic acid, folate, cobalamin, tocopherol or vitamin A each individually increases the toxicity of thalidomide and makes rats susceptible (Fratta *et al.*, 1965). Poor nutrition increases the half-life of most xenobiotics in the body.

21. Before and around the time of conception it is wise to avoid consuming food which has been overheated and contains appreciable amounts of the products of protein pyrolysis, which include some powerful mutagens that can increase the mutation rate of all body systems.

22. Men planning conception should have a good diet throughout the period of spermatogenesis. A poor diet or reduced food intake resulting from a loss of appetite or otherwise has been shown in animal experiments to increase mutation rate.

23. Women planning pregnancy should have the kind of diet associated with optimum birthweight and should avoid the restricted diet associated for example in the Hackney survey with low birthweight as shown in Table 5.6. Poor nutrition is a major risk factor for low birthweight. In the Hackney survey 28 mothers had babies with birthweights 2,500g and below and only one of these could be described as well fed and she had a low BMI. Now well-fed woman in the Hackney study had a baby who was growth-retarded in utero or small-for-dates. A recent paper from Sweden showed that 40 per cent of children with cerebral palsy had birthweights under 2,500g compared with 4.0 per cent in the general population (Hjalmasson *et al.*, 1988). An earlier Danish book on spastic cerebral palsy found 39 per cent of children with cerebral palsy had had low birthweights under 2,500g (Glenting, 1970). Papiernik (1978) quotes French figures suggesting that over 60 per cent of neurological handicap is associated with intrauterine growth retardation. In England and Wales 37 per cent of babies notified as having central nervous system malformations weighed under 2,500g at birth (OPCS, 1988). There are many other series showing low birthweight to be an indicator of about one half all congenital neurological handicap. As a corollary it may be inferred that about one half all neurological handicap is probably not caused by and is unconnected with maternal nutrition or low birthweight. Animal experiments have shown that mutations in male and female before conception can cause low birthweight and neurological disorders, and many of these mutations have causes unconnected with maternal nutrition.

PREVENTING THE REPETITION OF A DISAPPOINTING PREGNANCY

24. Couples anxious to prevent the repetition of a pregnancy which was a disappointment because of a miscarriage, a stillbirth, or because their baby

was of low birthweight, needed intensive care or was found to be handicapped, should be a priority for preconception care by the family doctor. A couple who have had a low birthweight baby should be offered nutritional counselling. Advice should be given on adequate spacing of the next pregnancy. A disappointing pregnancy is evidence of risk for any subsequent pregnancy. Following such a sad event a couple should be promised as part of postnatal care that help will be available if they wish to proceed with another pregnancy. Such couples should be referred for obstetric advice, for genetic counselling or to an appropriate specialist department (Chamberlain, 1990). Prepregnancy clinics have been established in London and their practice has been described (Chamberlain & Lumley, 1986). The French Ministry of Health recommended establishing clinics at major hospitals to help couples who have had a disappointing pregnancy (Mahon, 1972).

25. Care before conception can only reduce risks. Some handicap is still not preventible. But such is human suffering resulting from congenital handicap and chronic illness that care before conception is playing for very high stakes with very high penalties. There is a growing store of information on how risks can be reduced. Even small reductions in mutation rate and improvements in parental health will benefit some children.

References

Adams DD, Adams YJ, Knight JG, *et al.*, 1984. A solution to the genetic and environmental puzzles of insulin-dependent diabetes mellitus. *Lancet*; **i**: 420–4.

Adams JF, 1958. Pregnancy and Addisonian pernicious anaemia. *Scott Med J*; **3**: 21–5.

Adams PM, Fabricant JD, Legator MS, 1981. Cyclophosphamide-induced spermatogenic effects detected in the F_1 generation by behavioural testing. *Science*; **211**: 80–2.

Adler ID, 1982a. Germ-cell sensitivity in mammals. In: Sorsa M, Vainio H, eds. *Mutagens in our environment*. New York: Alan R Liss, 137–48.

Adler ID, 1982b. Male germ cell cytogenetics. In: Hsu TC, ed. *Cytogenetic assays of environmental mutagens*. Totowa NJ; Allanheld, 249–76.

Adler ID, 1982c. Mouse spermatogonia and spermatocyte sensitivity to chemical mutagens. *Cytogenet Cell Genet*; **33**: 95–100.

Adler ID, 1983a. Comparison of types of chemically induced genetic changes in mammals. *Mutat Res*; **115**: 293–321.

Adler ID, 1983b. Germ-cell sensitivity in mammals. *Mutat Res*; **113**: 221–327.

Alexander I, 1988. Chlamydia: one step forward or two backwards? *Br Med J*; **297**: 791.

Alink GM, Knize MG, Shen NH, Hesse SP, Felton JS, 1988. Mutagenicity of food pellets from human diets in Netherlands. *Mutat Res*; **206**: 387–93.

Alvarez OM, Gilbreath RL, 1982. Thiamine influence on collagen during the granulation of skin wounds. J Surg Res; **32**: 24–31.

Ames BN, 1983. Which are the significant mutagens and antimutagens? *Mutat Res*; **113**: 223–4.

Ames BN, McCann J, Yamasaki E, 1975. Methods for detecting carcinogens and mutagens with the salmonella/mammalian-microsome mutagenicity test. *Mutat Res*; **31**: 347–64.

Ando S, Rubens R, Rottiers R, 1984. Androgen plasma levels in male diabetics. *J Endocrinol Invest*; **7**: 21.

Arab L, Schellenberg B, Schlierf G, 1982. Nutrition and health; a survey of young men and women in Heidelberg. *Ann Nutr Metab*; **26** (suppl 1): 1–244.

Armstrong BK, Mann JI, Adelstein AM, Eskin F, 1975. Commodity consumption and ischaemic heart disease mortality with special reference to dietary practices. *J Chron Dis*; **28**: 455–69.

Arnold DL, Boyes BG, 1989. The toxicological effects of saccharin in short-term genotoxicity assays. *Mutat Res*; **221**: 69–132.

Astaldi G, Strosseli E, Airo R, 1962. Ricerche citogenitiche nelle emopatie: osservazioni sui cromosomi dell'anaemia perniciosa non trattata. *Boll Soc Ital Sper*; **38**: 111–4.

Auerbach C, Robson JM, 1946. Chemical production of mutations. *Nature*; **137**: 302–4.

Aula P, 1965. Virus-associated chromosome breakage. A cytogenetic study of chickenpox, measles and mumps patients and of cell cultures infected with measles virus. *Ann Acad Sci Fenn, A IV Biol*; **89**: 1–78.

Badr FM, Badr RS, 1975. Induction of dominant lethal mutation in male mice by alcohol. *Nature*; **253**: 133–6.

Badr FM, Rabouh SA, 1983. Effects of morphine sulphate on the germ cells of male mice. *Teratogenesis Carcinog Mutagen*; **3**: 19–26.

Badr FM, Rabouh SA, Badr RS, 1979. Mutagenicity of methadone hydrochloride induced dominant lethal mutation and spermatocyte chromosomal aberrations in treated males. *Mutat Res*; **68**: 235–49.

Baker R, Arlauskas A, Bonin A, Angus D, 1982. Detection of mutagenic activity in human urine following fried pork or bacon meals. *Cancer Lett*; **16**: 81–9.

Baker TG, 1982. Oogenesis and ovulation. In: Austin CR, Short RV, eds. *Reproduction in Mammals Book 1: Germ cells and fertilization.* Cambridge University Press, 17–45.

Bakke JL, Lawrence NL, Bennett J, Robinson S, 1975. Endocrine syndromes produced by neonatal hyperthyroidism, hypothyroidism, or altered nutrition and effects seen in untreated progeny. In: Fisher DA, Burrow GN, eds. *Perinatal Thyroid Physiology and Disease.* New York: Raven Press, 107–13.

Ballard JL, Holroyde J, Tsang RC, Chan G, Sutherland JM, Knowles HC, 1984. High malformation rates and decreased mortality in infants of diabetic mothers managed after the first trimester of pregnancy 1956–1978. *Am J Obstet Gynecol;* **148**: 1111–7.

Banduhn N, Obe G, 1985. Mutagenicity of methyl-2-benzimidazole carbamate, diethylstilbestrol and estradiol; structural chromosomal aberrations, sister-chromatid exchanges, C-mitoses polyploidies and micronuclei. *Mutat Res;* **156**: 199–218.

Baraitser M, 1983. Relevance of a family history of seizures. *Arch Dis Child;* **58**: 404–5.

Barale R, Zucconi D, Bertani R, Loprieno N, 1983. Vegetables inhibit, *in vivo*, the mutagenicity of nitrite combined with nitrosable compounds. *Mutat Res;* **120**: 145–50.

Barker DJP, Osmund C, 1986. Infant mortality, childhood nutrition, and ischaemic heart disease in England and Wales. *Lancet;* **i**: 1077–81.

Barker DJP, Winter PD, Osmund C, Margetts B, Simmonds SJ, 1989. Weight in infancy and death from ischaemic heart disease. *Lancet;* **ii**: 577–80.

Barlow SM, Sullivan FM, 1982. *Reproductive hazards of industrial chemicals.* London: Academic Press.

Barnes B, Bradley SG, 1990. *Planning for a healthy baby.* London: Ebury Press.

Barnett AH, Eff C, Leslie RDG, Pyke DA, 1981. Diabetes in identical twins: a study of 200 pairs. *Diabetologia;* **20**: 87–93.

Barnett G, Chiang CWN, 1983. Effects of marihuana on testosterone in male subjects. *J Theor Biol;* **104**: 685–92.

Bartak V, Josifko M, Horackova M, 1975. Juvenile diabetes and human sperm quality. *Int J Fertil;* **20**: 30–2.

Batzinger RP, Ou SYL, Bueding E, 1978. Antimutagenic effects of 2-tert-butyl-4-hydroxyanisole and antimicrobial agents. *Cancer Res;* **38**: 4478–85.

Beach RS, Gershwin ME, Hurley LS, 1982. Zinc, copper and manganese in immune function and experimental oncogenesis. *Nutr Cancer;* **3**: 172–91.

Beck L, Maier E, Schmidt E, Rohde J, 1978. *Mütter-und Säuglingssterblichkeit.* Stuttgart: Kohlhammer.

Becker K., Schöneich J, 1981. Effects of oestrogen on meiosis in female mice. *Mutat Res;* **85**: 226.

Beek B, Jacky PB, Sutherland GR, 1983. DNA precursor deprivation-induced chromosomal damage. *Mutat Res;* **113**: 331.

Belko AZ, Obarzanek E, Kalkwarf HJ, *et al.*, 1983. Effects of exercise on riboflavin requirements of young women. *Am J Clin Nutr;* **37**: 509–17.

Bell LT, Branstrator M, Roux C, Hurley LS, 1975. Chromosomal abnormalities in maternal and fetal tissues of magnesium and zinc-deficient rats. *Teratology;* **12**: 221–6.

Bell TA, 1985. Chlamydia trachomatis, mycoplasma hominis and ureaplasma urealyticum of infants. *Semin Perinatol;* **9**: 29–37.

Benda CE, 1949. Prenatal maternal factors in mongolism. *JAMA;* **139**: 979–85.

Bender MA, Preston RJ, 1982. Role of base damage in aberration formation. In: Natarajan AT, ed. *Progress in mutation research;* **4**: 37–46. Amsterdam: Elsevier.

Bennett PH, Webner C, Miller M, 1979. Congenital anomalies in the diabetic and pre-diabetic pregnancy. In: *Pregnancy metabolism, diabetes and the fetus.* Amsterdam: Excerpta Medica, 207–18. (Ciba Foundation Symposium 63)

Beral V, Roman E, Colwell L, 1984. Poor reproductive outcome in insulin-dependent diabetic women associated with later development of other endocrine disorders in the mothers. *Lancet;* **i**: 4–7.

van der Berg H, Schreurs WHP, Joosten GPA, 1978. Evaluation of the vitamin status in pregnancy. *Internat J Vitam Nutr Res*; **48**: 12–21.

Berg K, ed. 1979. *Genetic damage in man caused by environmental agents.* New York: Academic Press.

Bergh T, Nilhuis SJ, Wide L, 1978. Serum prolactin and gonadotrophin levels before and after luteinizing hormone-releasing hormone in the investigation of amenorrhoea. *Br J Obstet Gynaecol*; **85**: 945–6.

Bergstein NAM, 1979. *Pregnancy metabolism, diabetes and the fetus.* Amsterdam: Excerpta Medica, 275–6 (Ciba Foundation Symposium 63).

Bernhard P, 1962, Die Wirkung des Rauchens auf Frau und Mutter. *Muench Med Wochenschr*; **104**: 1826–8.

Bhatnagar A, Rani R, Ghosh PK, 1984. Chromosome aberrations and sister-chromatid exchanges (SCEs) in peripheral blood lymphocytes of patients suffering from poliomyelitis. *Mutat Res*; **141**: 55–8.

Bjeldanes LF, Morris MM, Felton J, *et al.*, 1982. Mutagens from the cooking of food; II survey by Ames/salmonella test of mutagen formation in the major protein-rich foods in the American diet. *Food Chem & Toxicol*; **20**: 357–63.

Bjelke E, 1975. Dietary vitamin A and human lung cancer. *Int J Cancer*; **15**: 561–5.

Bjelke E, 1978. Dietary factors and the epidemiology of cancer of the stomach and large bowel. *Aktuel Ernaehrungsmed Klin Prax: 2 (suppl)*: 10–7.

Bjerre B, Bjerre I, 1976. Significance of obstetric factors in prognosis of low birthweight children. *Acta Paediatr Scand*; **65**: 544–6.

Blake CA, Scaramuzzi RJ, Norman RL, Kanematsu S, Sawyer CH, 1972. Effect of nicotine on the proestrous ovulatory surge of LH in the rat. *Endocrinology*; **91**: 1253–8.

Blank H, 1986. *Papilloma viruses..* New York: John Wiley, 235. (Ciba Foundation Symposium 120).

Bleau G, Lemarbre J, Faucher G, Roberts KD, Chapdelaine A, 1984. Semen selenium and human fertility. *Fertil Steril*; **42**: 890–4.

Boas F, 1941. The relation between physical and mental development. *Science*; **93**: 339–42.

Bomsel-Helmreich O, Gougeon A, Thebault A, *et al.*, 1979. Healthy and atretic human follicles in the preovulatory phase. *J Clin Endocrinol Metab*; 48: 686-94.

Bonnar J, Redman CWG, Sheppard BL, 1975. Treatment of fetal growth and retardation in utero and dipyridamole. *Eur J Obstet Gynaecol Reprod Biol*; **5**: 123–34.

Bottura C, Coutinho V, 1967. The chromosome anomalies of the megaloblastic anaemias. *Blut*; **16**: 193–9.

Boué JG, Boué A, 1976. Chromosomal anomalies in early spontaneous abortions. In: Gropp A, Benirschke K, eds. *Developmental biology and pathology.* Heidelberg: Springer-Verlag, 193–208.

Boué JG, Boué A, Moorhead PS, Plotkin SA, 1964. Altérations chromosomiques induites par le virus de la rubéole dans les cellules embryonnaires diploides humaines cultivé *in vitro*. *CR Acad Sci*; **259**: 687–90.

Boué JG, Deluchat C, Nicolas H, Boué A, 1981a. Prenatal losses of trisomy 21. In: Burgio GR *et al.*, eds. *Trisomy 21.* Heidelberg; Springer-Verlag, -.

Boué JG, Deluchat C, Nicolas H, Boué A, 1981b. Prenatal losses of trisomy 21. *Hum Genet*; (suppl. 2): 183-93.

Brandriff B, Gordon L, Ashworth L, *et al.*, 1985. Chromosomes of human sperm: variability among normal individuals. *Hum Genet*; **70**: 18–24.

Bréart G, Rabarison Y, Plouin PF, Sureau C, Rumeau-Rouquette C, 1982. Risk of fetal growth retardation as a result of maternal hypertension. *Dev Pharmacol Ther*; **4** (suppl. 1): 116–23.

Brewen JG, Payne HS, 1979. X-ray stage sensitivity of mouse oocytes and its bearing on dose-response curves. *Genetics*; **91**: 149–51.

Brewen JG, Payne HS, Jones KP, Preston RT, 1975. Studies on chemically induced dominant lethality; the cytogenetic basis of MMS-induced dominant lethality in post-meiotic male germ cells. *Mutat Res*; **33**: 239–50.

Brewen JG, Payne HS, Preston RT, 1976. X-ray induced chromosome aberrations in mouse dictyate oocytes: I time and dose relationships. *Mutat Res*; **35**: 111–20.

Bridges BA, 1987. Alcohol as a mutagenic agent. *Mutat Res*; **186**: 173–6.

Bridges BA, Clemmesen J, Sugimura T, 1979. Cigarette smoking – does it carry a genetic risk? *Mutat Res*; **65**: 71–81.

Briggs MH, 1973. Cigarette smoking and infertility in men. *Med J Aust*; **i**: 616.

Brown GM, Garfinkel PE, Jeuniwic N, Moldofsky H, Stancer HC, 1977. Endocrine profiles in anorexia nervosa. In: Vigersky RA, ed. *Anorexia nervosa*. New York: Raven Press, 123–35.

Bruce WR, Varghese AJ, Wang S, Dion P, 1979. The endogenous production of nitroso compounds in the colon and cancer at that site. In: Miller EC *et al.*, eds. *Naturally occurring carcinogens-mutagens and modulation of carcinogenesis*. Baltimore, University Park Press, 221–8.

Brusick D, 1980. *Principles of genetic toxicology*. New York: Plenum Press.

Bryce-Smith D, 1985. *Elemental nutrients and antinutrients in prenatal development*. First Symposium on Preconception Care. Maidenhead: Wyeth, 10–3.

Bryce-Smith D, 1986. Environmental chemical influences on behaviour and mentation. *Chem Soc Rev*; **15**: 93–123.

Bryce-Smith D, Deshpande R.R., Hughes T, Waldron HA, 1977. Lead and cadmium in stillbirths. *Lancet*; **i**: 1159.

Buckton KE, 1983. Incidence and some consequences of X-chromosome abnormalities in liveborn infants. In: Sandberg AA, ed. *Chromosome anomalies and their clinical manifestations*. New York: Alan Liss, 7–22.

Burger EJ, Tardiff RG, Scialli AR, Zenick H, 1989. *Sperm measures and reproductive success.* New York; Alan Liss.

Burger GCE, Drummond JC, Sandstead HR, eds., 1948. *Malnutrition and Starvation in Western Netherlands; September 1944 to July 1945*. The Hague: General State Printing Office.

Burke BS, 1948. Nutritional needs in pregnancy in relation to nutritional intakes as shown in dietary histories. *Obstet Gynecol Surv*; **3**: 716–27.

Burke BS, Harding VV, Stuart HC, 1943. Nutrition studies during pregnancy. *J Pediatr*; **23**: 506–15.

Burke BS, Stevenson SS, Worcester J, Stuart HC, 1949. Nutrition studies during pregnancy: V Relation of maternal nutrition to condition of infant at birth: study of siblings. *J Nutr*; **38**: 453–67.

Busch E, 1954. Versuche zur Beinflussung von Bullensperma durch Vitamin B12. Dissertation. Tierärztliche Hochschule, Hannover. *Animal Breeding Abstracts*; **25**: 44, No. 147, 1957.

Butcher RL, 1981. Experimentally induced gametopathies. In: Iffy L, Kaminetzky HA, eds. *Principles and Practice of Obstetrics and Perinatology*. New York: John Wiley, 339–49.

Butcher RL, Fugo NW, 1967. Overripeness and the mammalian ova: II Delayed ovulation and chromosomal anomalies. *Fertil Steril*; **18**: 297.

Butcher RL, Pope RS, 1979. Role of estrogen during prolonged estrous cycles of the rat on subsequent embryonic death or development *Biol Reprod*; **21**: 491–5.

Butcher RL, 1976. Pre-ovulatory and post-ovulatory overripeness. *Int J Gynaecol Obst*; **14**: 105–10.

Caan B, Horgen DM, Margen S, King JC, Jewell NP, 1987. Benefits associated with WIC supplemental feeding during the interpregnancy interval. *Am J Clin Nutr*; **45**: 29–41.

Calabrese LH, Kirkendall DT, Floyd M, *et al.*, 1983. Menstrual abnormalities, nutritional patterns and body composition in female classical ballet dancers. *Physiol Sports Med*; **11**: 86–98.

Callard IP, Leathem JH, 1970. Pregnancy maintenance in protein deficient rats. *Acta Endocrinol (Copenh)*; **63**: 544–559.

Canada, 1975. *Nutrition Canada: Quebec*. Ottawa: Department of Health and Welfare.

Carr DH, 1970. Chromosome abnormalities and spontaneous abortions. In: Jacobs PA, Price WH, Law P, eds. *Human population cytogenetics*. Edinburgh University Press, 103–18.

Cattanach BM, 1966a. Chemically induced mutations in mice. *Mutat Res*; **3**: 346–53.

Cattanach BM, 1966b. Induction of paternal sex-chromosome losses and deletions and of autosomal gene mutations by the treatment of mouse post-meiotic germ cells with triethylenemelamine. *Mutat Res*; **4**: 73–82.

Cattanach BM, 1982. Induction of specific-locus mutations in female mice by triethylenemelamine (TEM). *Mutat Res*; **104**: 173–6.

Chamberlain G, 1986. Prepregnancy care. In: Chamberlain G, Lumley J, eds. *Prepregnancy care: a manual for practice*. New York: John Wiley, 1–10.

Chamberlain G, 1990. Preparing for pregnancy: a health primer for parents-to-be. London: Fontana.

Chamberlain G, Lumley J, eds. 1986. *Prepregnancy care: a manual for practice*. New York: John Wiley.

Chamberlain G, Philipp E, Howlett B, Masters K, 1978. *British Births 1970*: vol 2 obstetric care. London: Heinemann.

Chamberlain R, Chamberlain G, Howlett B, Claireaux A, 1975. *British Births 1970*: vol. 1 The first week of life. London: Heinemann.

Chamberlin J, Magenis RE, 1980. Parental origin of de novo chromosome rearrangements. *Hum Genet*; **53**: 343–7.

Chandra RK, ed. 1988. *Nutrition and immunology*. New York: Alan Liss.

Chang MW, Choi TK, Matsuo Y, Yoshii Z, 1984. Influence of ureaplasma urealyticum and mycoplasma hominis on the human spermatozoal motility. *Hiroshima J Med Sci*; **33**: 23–6.

Charles D, Finland M, 1973. *Obstetric and perinatal infections*. Philadelphia: Lea & Febiger.

Cheek DB, Graystone J, Mehrizi A, 1966. The importance of muscle cell number in children with heart disease. *Bull Johns Hopkins Hosp*; **118**: 140–50.

Chieri RA, Rivetta OM, Foglia VG, 1969. Altered ovulation pattern in experimental diabetes. *Fertil Steril*; **20**: 661–6.

Chu EHY, Generoso WM, 1983, eds. *Mutation, cancer and malformations*. New York: Plenum Press.

Chung C, Myrionthopoulos WC, 1975. Effect of maternal diabetes on congenital malformations. *National Foundation March of Dimes, Original article series*; **11**: 23–8.

Cicero TJ, 1982. Alcohol-induced deficits in the hypothalamic-pituitary-luteinizing hormone axis in the male. *Alcoholism (NY)*; **6**: 207–15.

Cicero TJ, Meyer ER, Bell PD, 1979. Effect of ethanol on the hypothalamic-pituitary-luteinizing hormone axis and testicular steroidogenesis. *J Pharmacol Exp Ther*; **208**: 210–15.

Clermont Y, Bustos-Obregon E, 1968. Re-examination of spermatogonial renewal in the rat by means of seminiferous tubules mounted "*in toto*". *Am J Anat*; **122**: 237–48.

Clermont Y, Hermo L, 1975. Spermatogonial stem cells in the albino rat. *Am J Anat*; **142**: 159–76.

Commoner B, Vithayathil AJ, Polasa P, Nair S, Madyastha P, Cuca GC, 1978. Formation of mutagens in beef and beef extract during cooking. *Science*; **201**: 913.

Coop IE, 1966. Effect of flushing on reproductive performance of ewes. *J Agric Sci (Camb)*; **67**: 305–23.

Courot M, 1982. Facteurs masculins de la fertilité; apports et limites des études chez l'animal. In: Spira A, Jouannet P, eds. *Les facteurs de la fertilité humaine*. Paris: INSERM, 45–56.

Cox BD, Lyon MF, 1975. X-ray induced dominant lethal mutations in mature and immature oocytes of guinea-pigs and golden hamsters. *Mutat Res*; **28**: 421–36.

Cruickshanks KJ, Dorman JS, Aarons J, *et al.*, 1984. Pregnancy outcome in diabetics with other endocrine disorders. *Lancet*; **i**: 629–30.

Dansky LD, Andermann E, Andermann F, 1980. Marriage and fertility in epileptic patients. *Epilepsia*; **21**: 261–71.

David G, 1982. Facteurs de variation des caractéristiques du sperme. In: Spira A, Jouannet P, eds. *Les facteurs de la fertilité humaine*. Paris: INSERM; **57**: 67.

Decker K, Hinselmann M, Glatzle D, 1975. Anämie und Schwangerschaft. In: Brubacher G, Ritzel G, eds. *Zur Ernährungssituation der schweizerischen Bevölkerung*. Bern: Hans Huber; 221–32.

Dinsdale D, Williams RB, 1980. Ultrastructural changes in the sperm-tail of zinc-deficient rats. *Journal of Comparative Pathology*; **90**: 559–66.

Dion PW, Brightsee ER, Smith CC, Bruce WR, 1982. The effect of dietary ascorbic acid and alpha-tocopherol on fecal mutagenicity. *Mutat Res*; **102**: 27-37.

Distiller LA, Sagel J, Morley JE, Joffe BI, Seftel HC, 1975. Pituitary responsiveness to luteinizing hormone-releasing hormone in insulin-dependent diebetes mellitus. *Diabetes*; **24**: 378-80.

Dizerega GS, Hodgen GD, 1981. Luteal phase dysfunction infertility: a sequel to aberrant folliculogenesis. *Fertil Steril*; **35**: 489–99.

Dorfler R, Voigt A, 1966. Virus hepatitis and pregnancy, frequency and reciprocal influence. *Muench Med Wochenschr*; **108**: 1042.

Doyle W, Crawford MA, Lawrence BM, Drury P, 1982. Dietary survey during pregnancy in a low socio-economic group. *Hum Nutr: Appl Nutr*; **36A**: 95–106.

Doyle W, Crawford MA, Wynn AHA, Wynn SW, 1989a. Maternal magnesium intake and pregnancy outcome. *Magnesium Res*; **2**: 205–10.

Doyle W, Crawford MA, Wynn AHA, Wynn SW, 1989b. Maternal nutrient intake and birthweight. *J Hum Nutr Diet*; **2**: 415–22.

Doyle W, Crawford MA, Wynn AHA, Wynn SW, 1990. The association of maternal diet and birth dimensions. *J Nutr Med*; **1**: 9–16.

Dunn HG, Hughes CJ, Schulzer M, 1986. Physical growth. In: Dunn HG, ed. *Sequelae of low birthweight: The Vancouver Study*. Clinics in Developmental Medicine No. 95/96. Oxford: Blackwell, 35–53.

Eckhert CD, Hurley LS, 1977. Reduced DNA synthesis in zinc deficiency: regional differences in embryonic rats. *J Nutr*; **107**: 855–61.

Edwards RG, Steptoe PC, 1975. Induction of follicular growth ovulation and luteinization in the human ovary. *J Reprod Fertil*; **22** (suppl): 121–63.

Ehling UH, 1971. Comparison of radiation- and chemically- induced dominant lethal mutations in male mice. *Mutat Res*; **11**: 35–44.

Ehling UH, 1979. Induction of dominant lethal mutations in male mice by fosfestrol. *Arch Toxicol*; **42**: 171–7.

Ehling UH, Neuhäuser-Klaus A, 1988. Induction of specific locus and dominant lethal mutations by cyclophosphamide and combined cyclophosphamide radiation treatment in male mice. *Mutat Res*; **199**: 21–30.

Ejima Y, Sasaki MS, Kaneko A, Tanooka H, 1988. Types, rates, origin and expressivity of chromosome mutations involving 13q14 in retinoblastoma patients. *Hum Genet*; **79**: 118–23.

Ek JI, 1959. Thyroid function in mothers of mongoloid infants. *Acta Paediatr Scand*; **48**: 33–42.

Emerit I, Emerit J, Levy A, Kech M, 1979. Chromosomal breakage in Crohn's disease: anticlastogenic effect of D-penicillamine and L cysteine. *Hum Genet*; **50**: 51–7.

Emerit I, Emerit J, Tosoni-Pittoni A, Bousquet O, Sarrazin A, 1972. Chromosome studies in patients with ulcerative colitis. *Humangenetik*; **16**: 313–22.

Emerit I, Feingold J, Camus J, Housset E, 1974. Étude chromosomique des maladies du collagène. *Ann Génét (Paris)*; **17**: 251–6.

Emerit I, Marteau R, 1971. Chromosome studies in 14 patients with disseminated sclerosis. *Humangenetik*; **13**: 25–33.

EMIC-UK, The Environmental Mutagen Information Centre, United Kingdom Office, University College, Swansea.

Endo A, 1966. Teratogenesis in diabetic mice treated with alloxan prior to conception. *Arch Environ Health*; **12**: 492–500.

Endo A, Ingalls TH, 1968. Chromosomal anomalies in embryos of diabetic mice. *Arch Environ Health*; **16**: 316–25.

Epstein SS, Arnold E, Andrea J, Bass W, Bishop Y, 1972. Detection of chemical mutagens by the dominant lethal assay in the mouse. *Toxicol Appl Pharmacol*; **23**: 288.

Epstein SS, Röhrborn G, 1970. Recommended procedures for testing genetic hazards from chemicals, based on the induction of dominant lethal mutations in mammals. *Nature*; **230**: 459–60.

Esch MW, Easter RA, Bahr JM, 1981. Effect of riboflavine deficiency on estrous cyclicity in pigs. *Biol Reprod*; **25**: 659–65.

European Environmental Mutagen Society, 1978. Mutagenicity screening: general principles and minimal criteria. *Mutat Res*; **53**: 361–7.

European Environmental Mutagen Society, 1983. Estimation of genetic risks and increased incidence of genetic disease due to environmental mutagens. *Mutat Res*; **115**: 255–91.

Evered D, Clark S, eds. 1986. *Papillomaviruses*. New York: John Wiley. (Ciba Foundation Symposium 120)

Fairburn CG, McCulloch DK, Wu FC, 1982. The effects of diabetes on male sexual function. *Clin Endocrinol Metab*; **11**: 749–67.

Fenech M, Morley AA, 1985. The effect of donor age on spontaneous and induced micronuclei. *Mutat Res*; **148**: 99–105.

Fialkow PJ, Thuline HC, Hecht F, Bryant J, 1971. Familial predisposition to thyroid disease in Down's syndrome: controlled immunoclinical studies. *Am J Hum Genet*; **23**: 67–86.

Field B, Kerr C, 1981. Season and interval for recurrence of neural tube defects. *J Med Genet*; **18**: 484.

Finland M, 1973. Influenza complicating pregnancy. In: Charles D, Finland M, eds. *Obstetric and Perinatal Infections*. Philadelphia: Lee & Febiger, 355–98.

Fletcher AC, 1985. Reproductive hazards at work. Manchester: Equal Opportunities Commission.

Forbes AP, Engel E, 1963. The high incidence of diabetes mellitus in 41 patients with gonadal dysgenesis, and their close relatives. *Metabolism*; **12**: 428–39.

Foresight: Association for the Promotion of Pre-Conceptual Care, 1985. *Guidelines for future parents*. Old Vicarage, Church Lane, Godalming, Surrey GU8 5PN.

Forteza BG, Baguena RC, 1963. Analisis citogenetico de un caso de anemia pernicioso antes y despues del tratamiento. *Rev Clin Esp*; **88**: 251–54.

Fox BW, Jackson H, Craig AW, Glover TD, 1963. Effects of alkylating agents on spermatogenesis in the rabbit. *J Reprod Fertil*; **5**: 13–22.

Fratta ID, Sigg EB, Maiorana K, 1965. Teratogenic effect of thalidomide in rabbits, rats, hamsters and mice. *Toxicol Appl Pharmacol*; **7**: 268–86.

Freed JJ, Schatz SA, 1969. Chromosomal aberrations in cultured cells deprived of single essential amino acids. *Exp Cell Res*; **55**: 393–409.

Friedman JM, 1981. Genetic disease in the offspring of older fathers. *Obstet Gynecol*; **57**: 745–9.

Fries H, 1974. Secondary amenorrhoea and self-induced weight reduction and anorexia nervosa. *Acta Psychiat Scand*; **50** (suppl 248).

Frisch RE, 1977. Food intake, fatness and reproductive ability. In: Vigersky RA, ed. *Anorexia nervosa*. New York: Raven Press, 139–61.

Fuhrmann K, Reiher H, Semmler K, Fischer F, Fischer M, Glockner E, 1983. Prevention of congenital malformations in infants of insulin-dependent diabetic mothers. *Diabetes Care*; **6**: 219–23.

Furuhjelm M, Jonson B, Lagergren CG, 1962. The quality of human semen in spontaneous abortion. *Int J Fertil*; **7**: 17–21.

Gardner MJ, Snee MP, Hall AJ, Powell CA, Downs S, Terrel JD, 1990. Results of case-control study of leukaemia and lymphoma among young people near Sellafield nuclear plant in West Cumbria. *Br Med J*; **300**: 423–9.

Gates AH, Donaldson CH, Levy MD, 1981. Oocyte aneuploidy screening using superovulating prepubertal mice: effect of methotrexate. *Teratology*; **24**: 321–7.

Gavaler JS, Van Thiel DH, 1987. Reproductive consequences of alcohol abuse: males and females compared and contrasted. *Mutat Res*; **186**: 269–77.

Gellis SS, Hsia Y-YD, 1959. The infant of the diabetic mother. *Am J Dis Child*; **97**: 1–41.

Gelpi AP, 1970. Fatal hepatitis in Saudi Arabian women. *Am J Gastroenterol*; **53**: 41.

Generoso WM, 1969. Chemical induction of dominant lethals in female mice. *Genetics*; **61**: 461–70.

Generoso WM, 1983. Dominant lethal mutations and heritable translocations in mice. In: Chu EHY, Generoso WM, eds. *Mutation, cancer and malformations.* New York: Plenum Press, 369–88.

Generoso WM, Cain KT, Cornett CC, Cacheiro NLA, 1984. DNA target sites associated with chemical inducation of dominant-lethal mutations and heritable translocations in mice. In: Chopra VL, Joshi RP *et al.*, eds. *Genetics: new frontiers.* Oxford University Press, 347–55.

Generoso WM, Rutledge JC, Cain KT, Hughes LA, Braden PW, 1987. Exposure of female mice to ethylene oxide within hours after mating leads to fetal malformation and death. *Mutat Res*; **176**: 269–74.

Generoso WM, Rutledge JC, Cain KT, Hughes LA, Downing DJ, 1988. Mutation-induced fetal anomalies and death following treatment of females within hours after mating. *Mutat Res*; **199**: 175–81.

Gershenson SM, 1986. Viruses as environmental mutagenic factors. *Mutat Res*; **167**: 203–13.

Ghosh R, Ghosh PK, 1983. Sister-chromatid exchanges in herpes simplex infection. *Mutat Res*; **117**: 303–8.

Giroud A, Lefèbvres-Boisselot J, 1951. Anomalies provoquées chez le foetus en l'absence d'acide folique. *Arch Fr Pédiatr*; **8**: 648–56.

Giroud A, Ettori J, Boisselot J, 1949. Déficience en riboflavine chez la rate à la limite permittant la gestation. *Int Z Vitaminforsch*; **21**: 261–5.

Giroud A, Levy G, Lefèbvres-Boisselot J, 1950. Taux de la riboflavine chez le foetus de rat présentant des malformations dues à la déficience B2. *Int Z Vitaminforsch*; **22**: 308–12.

Giroud A, Levy G, Lefèbvres J, Dupuis R, 1952. Chute du taux de la riboflavine au stade où se déterminent les malformations embryonnaires. *Int Z Vitaminforsch*; **23**: 490–4.

Giroud A, Tuchmann-Duplessis H, Mercier-Parot L, 1962. Observations sur les répercussions tératogenes de la thalidomide chez la souris et le lapin. *CR Soc Biol (Paris)*; **156**: 765–8.

Glenting P, 1970. *Etiology of congenital spastic cerebral palsy.* Copenhagen: FADLs Forlag.

Goldstein S, 1978. Human genetic disorders that feature premature onset and accelerated progression of biological aging. In: Schneider EL, ed. *The genetics of ageing.* New York: Plenum Press, 171–224.

Gontzea J, 1965. *Die richtige Ernährung der schwangeren und der stillenden Frau und ihre Bedeutung für die Gesundheit von Mutter und Kind.* Jena: Fischer Verlag.

Green S, Auletta A, Fabricant J, Kapp R, *et al.*, 1985. Current status of bioassays in genetic toxicology – the dominant lethal assay. *Mutat Res*; **154**: 49–67.

Greenwood M, 1928. 'Laws' of mortality from the biological point of view. *J Hyg*; **28**: 267–94.

Gross SJ, Kosmetatos N, Grimes CT, Williams ML, 1978. Newborn head size and neurological status. *Am J Dis Child*; **132**: 753–6.

de Grouchy J, 1970. 21p-maternel en double exemplaire chez un trisomique 21. *Ann Génét*; **13**: 52–5.

Gubler CJ, 1982. Thiamin: 20 years of progress. *Ann NY Acad Sci*; **378**: 440.

Gunn SA, Gould TC, 1957. Hormone interrelationships affecting the selective uptake of ^{65}Zn by the dorso-lateral prostate of the hypophysectomized rat. *J Endocrinol*; **16**: 18–27.

Habibzadek N, Schorah CJ, Smithells RW, 1986. The effects of maternal folic acid and vitamin C nutrition in early pregnancy on reproductive performance in the guinea-pig. *Brit J Nutr*; **55**: 23–35.

Hale F, 1933. Pigs born without eyeballs. *J Hered*; **24**: 105–6.

Halkka O, Halkka L, 1969. Induction of chromosome aberrations in spermatogenesis by intracellular microbes. *Chromosomes Today*; **2**: 61–9.

Hall M, Davidson RJL, 1968. Prophylactic folic acid in women with pernicious anaemia pregnant after periods of infertility. *J. Clin Path*; **21**: 599–602.

Hamfelt A, Tuvemo T, 1972. Pyridoxal phosphate and folic acid concentration in blood and erythrocyte aspartate aminotransferase activity during pregnancy. *Clin Chim Acta*; **41**: 287–98.

Hampar B, Ellison SA, 1961. Chromosomal aberrations induced by an animal virus. *Nature*; **192**: 145–7.

Hansmann I, 1984. Aspects of nondisjunction. In: Obe G, ed. *Mutations in man.* Heidelberg: Springer-Verlag, 147-55.

Hardy JB, Azarowicz EN, Mannini A, Medearis DN, Cooke RE, 1961. The effect of Asian influenza on the outcome of pregnancy, Baltimore 1957-58. *Am J Public Health;* **51**: 1182–8.

Haresign W, Cole DJA, 1981. *Recent Developments in ruminant nutrition.* London: Butterworth.

Harlap S, Shiono PH, 1980. Alcohol, smoking and incidence of spontaneous abortions in the 1st and 2nd trimester. *Lancet;* **ii**: 173–76.

Harper MJK, 1982. Sperm and egg transport. In: Austin CR, Short RV, eds. *Reproduction in mammals Book 1: Germ cells and fertilization.* Cambridge University Press: 102–27.

Harris JW, 1919. Influenza occurring in pregnant women. A statistical study of thirteen hundred and fifty cases. *JAMA;* **72**: 978.

Hatanaka Y, Ueda K, 1981. High incidence of subclinical hypovitaminosis of B1 among university students found by a field study in Ehime, Japan. *Med J Osaka Univ;* **31**: 83–91.

Hayatsu H, Arminoto S, Togawa K, Makita M, 1981a. Inhibitory effect of the ether extract of human feces on activities of mutagens: inhibition by oleic and linoleic acids. *Mutat Res;* **81**: 287–93.

Hayatsu H, Inoue K, Ohta H, *et al.*, 1981b. Inhibition of the mutagenicity of cooked beef basic fraction by its acidic fraction. *Mutat Res;* **91**: 437–42.

Hayatsu H, Hayatsu T, Ohara Y, 1985. Mutagenicity of human urine caused by ingestion of fried ground beef. *Jpn J Cancer Res;* **76**: 445–8.

Hayatsu H, Arminoto S, Negishi T, 1988. Dietary inhibitors of mutagenesis and carcinogenesis. *Mutat Res;* **202**: 429–46.

Heap RB, Flint APF, 1984. Pregnancy. In: Austin CR, Short RV, eds. *Reproduction in Mammals; Book 3 Hormonal control of reproduction.* Cambridge University Press, 153–94.

Heath CW, 1966. Cytogenetic observations in vitamin B12 and folate deficiency. *Blood;* **27**: 800–15.

Hecht F, Hecht BK, 1984. Fragile sites and chromosome breakpoints in constitutional rearrangements: II Spontaneous abortions, stillbirths and newborns. *Clin Genet;* **26**: 174–77.

Heller CG, Clermont Y, 1964. Kinetics of the germinal epithelium in man. *Recent Prog Horm Res;* **20**: 545–71.

Herrmann J, 1966. Der Einfluß des Zeugungsalters auf die Mutationen zu Hämophilie A. *Humangenetik;* **3**: 1–16.

Hertig AT, 1967. Human trophoblast: normal and abnormal. *Am J Clin Pathol;* **47**: 249–70.

Hertig AT, Sheldon WH, 1943. Minimal criteria required to prove prima facie case of traumatic abortion or miscarriage. *Ann Surg;* **117**: 595–606.

Hirvonen E, 1977. Etiology, clinical features and prognosis in secondary amenorrhoea. *Int J Fertil;* **22**: 69–76.

Hjalmasson O, Hagberg B, Hagberg G, 1988. Epidemiologic panorama of brain impairments and causative factors: Swedish experiences. In: Kubli F *et al.*, eds. *Perinatal events and brain damage in surviving children.* Heidelberg: Springer-Verlag, 28–36.

Hongslo JK, Christensen T, Brunborg G, Bjornstad C, Holme JA, 1988. Genotoxic effects of paracetamol in V79 Chinese hamster cells. *Mutat Res;* **204**: 333–41.

Hook EB, 1982. Contribution of chromosome abnormalities to human morbidity and mortality. *Cytogenet Cell Genet;* **33**: 101–6.

Hook, EB, Schreinmachers DM, Willey AM, Cross PK, 1984. Inherited structural cytogenetic abnormalities detected incidentally to fetuses diagnosed prenatally: frequency, parental-age associations, sex-ratio trends and comparisons with rates of mutants. *Am J Hum Genet;* **36**: 422–43.

Howell WH, 1890. The life-history of the formed elements of the blood, especially the red corpuscles. *J Morphol;* **4**: 57.

Howland BE, 1975. The influence of feed restriction and subsequent refeeding on gonadotrophin secretion and serum testosterone levels in male rats. *J Reprod Fertil;* **44**: 429–36.

Ho-Yen DO, Joss AWL, 1988. Toxoplasma and cytomegalovirus infections during pregnancy. *Matern Child Health;* **13**: 225–7.

Hsu TC, Liang JC, Shirley LR, 1983. Aneuploidy induction by mitotic arrestants; effects of diazepam on diploid Chinese hamster cells. *Mutat Res*; **122**: 201–9.

Huang HFS, Dyrenfurth I, Hembree WC, 1983. Endocrine changes associated with germ cell loss during vitamin A-induced recovery of spermatogenesis. *Endocrinology*; **112**: 1163–71.

Huang HFS, Marshall GR, 1983. Failure of spermatid release under various vitamin A states – an indication of delayed spermiation. *Biol Reprod*; **28**: 1163–72.

Hugenholtz AP, Bruce WR, 1976. Induction and transmission of elevated levels of abnormally shaped murine sperm. *Can J Genet Cytol*; **18**: 564.

Hurley LS, 1979. Nutritional deficiencies and excesses. In: Wilson JG, Fraser FC, eds. *Handbook of teratology*. New York: Plenum Press, 261–308.

Hurley LS, 1981. Teratogenic aspects of manganese, zinc and copper nutrition. *Physiol Rev*; **61**: 249–95.

Hurley R, 1983. Virus infections in pregnancy and the puerperium. In: Waterson AP, ed. *Recent advances in clinical virology*. Edinburgh: Churchill Livingstone, 19–55.

Hutchinson HE, Ferguson-Smith MA, 1959. The significance of Howell-Jolly bodies in red cell precursors. *J Clin Pathol*; **12**: 451–3.

ICPEMC; International Commission for Protection against Environmental Mutagens and Carcinogens, 1979. Cigarette smoking – does it carry a genetic risk? *Mutat Res*; **65**: 71–81.

ICPEMC; International Commission for Protection against Environmental Mutagens and Carcinogens, 1983. Estimation of genetic risks and increased incidence of genetic disease due to environmental mutagens. *Mutat Res*; **115**: 255–91.

ICPEMC; International Commission for Protection against Environmental Mutagens and Carcinogens, 1986. Inhibitors of mutagenesis and their relevance to carcinogenesis: report by expert group on antimutagens and desmutagens. *Mutat Res*; **168**: 47–68.

Iffy L, 1981. The concept of the aging ovum. In: Iffy L, Kaminetzky, HA eds. *Principles and Practice of Obstetrics and Perinatology*, New York: John Wiley, 323–37.

Iivanainen M, 1974. *A study on the origins of mental retardation*. London: Heinemann. (Clinics in Developmental Medicine 51)

Im MJC, Freshwater MF, Hoopes JE, 1975. Enzyme activities in granulation tissue; energy for collagen synthesis. *J Surg Res*; **20**: 121–5.

Ivanov B, Léonard A, Deknudt G, 1973. Blood storage and the rate of chromosome aberrations after in vivo exposure to ionizing radiations. *Radiat Res*; **55**: 469–76.

Itokawa Y, Sasagawa S, Fujiwara M, 1973. Effects of thiamine on lipid metabolism in magnesium deficient rats. *J Nutr Sci Vitaminol (Tokyo)*; **19**: 15–21.

Itokawa Y, Tseng LF, Fujiwara M, 1974. Thiamine metabolism in magnesium-deficient rats. *J Nutr Sci Vitaminol (Tokyo)*; **20**: 249–55.

Jacky PB, Beek B, Sutherland GR, 1983. Fragile sites in chromosomes: possible model for the study of spontaneous chromosome breakage. *Science*; **220**: 69–70.

Jagiello G, 1981. Reproduction in Down's syndrome. In: de la Cruz FF, Gerald PS, eds. *Trisomy 21 (Down's syndrome)*. Baltimore: University Park Press, 151–62.

Janz D, Beck-Mannagetta G, Scheffner D, Scholz G, 1982. Epilepsy in children of epileptic parents. In: Janz D, *et al.*, eds. *Epilepsy, Pregnancy and the Child*. New York: Raven Press, 527–534.

Jolly J, 1905. Sur la formation des globules rouges des mammifères. *CR Soc Biol (Paris)*; **57**: 528–31.

Jones KL, Smith DW, Harvey MAS, Hall BD, Quan L, 1975. Old paternal age and fresh gene mutation: Data on additional disorders. *J Pediatr*; **86**: 84–8.

Jongbloet PH, 1986. Prepregnancy care: background biological effects. In Chamberlain G, Lumley J, eds. *Prepregnancy care: a manual for practice*. New York: John Wiley, 31–52.

Jouannet P, Ducot B, Soumah A, Spira A, Feneux D, Albert M, 1981. Les caractéristiques du sperme des hommes féconds et inféconds. In: Spira A, Jouannet P, eds. *Les facteurs de la fertilité humaine*. Paris: INSERM, 73–89.

Juberg RC, Mowrey PN, 1983. Origin of nondisjunction in trisomy 21 syndrome. *Am J Med Genet*; **16**: 111–6.

Kada T, 1982. Mechanisms and genetic implications of environmental antimutagens. In: Sugimura T, Kondo S, Takebe H, eds. *Environmental mutagens and carcinogens.* New York: Alan Liss, 355–9.

Kada T, Marita K, Inoue T, 1978. Antimutagenic action of vegetable factor(s) on the mutagenic principle of tryptophan pyrolysate. *Mutat Res*; **53**: 351–3.

Kada T, Kaneko K, Matsuzaki S, Matsuzaki T, Hara Y, 1985. A case of the green tea factor. *Mutat Res*; **150**: 127–32.

Kalimo K, Teho P, Honkonen E, Grönroos M, Halonen P, 1981. Chlamydia trachomatis and herpes simplex virus IgA antibodies in cervical secretions of patients with cervical atypia. *Br J Obstet Gynaecol*; **88**: 1130–4.

Kalla NR, 1981. Effect of vitamin A deficient diet on the spermatogenesis and plasma testosterone. *Acta Europe Fertil*; **12**: 249–253.

Kamiguchi Y, Funaki K, Mikamo K, 1979. Chromosomal anomalies caused by preovulatory overripeness of the primary oocyte. *Proc Jpn Acad*; **55 B**: 398–402.

Kaminetzky HA, Langer A, Baker H, et al, 1973. The effect of nutrition in teenage pregnancy and the status of the neonate. *Am J Obstet Gynecol*; **115**: 639–46.

Karp LE, 1980. Older fathers and genetic mutations. *Am J Hum Genet*; **7**: 405–6.

Katoh M, Cacheiro NLA, Cornett CV, Cain KT, Rutledge JC, Generoso WM, 1989. Fetal anomalies produced subsequent to treatment of zygotes with ethylene oxide or ethyl methanesulfonate are not likely due to the usual genetic causes. *Mutat Res*; **210**: 337–44.

Kaufman MH, 1982. The chromosome complement of single-pronuclear haploid mouse embryos following activation by ethanol treatment. *J Embryol Exp Morphol*; **71**: 139–54.

Kaufman MH, 1983. Ethanol-induced chromosomal abnormalities at conception. *Nature*; **302**: 258–60.

Kaufman MH, 1985. An hypothesis regarding the origin of aneuploidy in man: indirect evidence from an experimental model. *J Med Genet*; **22**: 171–8.

Kato H, Sandberg AA, 1977. Effects of herpes simplex virus on sister chromatid exchanges and chromosome abnormalities in human diploid fibroblasts. *Exp Cell Res*; **109**: 423–7.

Kendall EJC, 1985. Acute respiratory infections in the population. *J R Soc Med*; **78**: 282–90.

Kibrick S, 1973. Herpes Simplex. In: Charles D, Finland M, eds. *Obstetric and perinatal infections.* Philadephia: Lea & Febiger, 75–94.

Kinzey WG, Srebnik HH, 1963. Maintenance of pregnancy in protein-deficient rats with short-term injections of ovarian hormones. *Proc Soc Exp Biol Med*; **114**: 158–60.

Kiossoglou KA, Mitus WJ, Dameshek W, 1965. Chromosomal aberrations in pernicious anemia. Study of three cases before and after therapy. *Blood*; **25**: 662.

Kirk KM, Lyon MF, 1982. Induction of congenital anomalies in offspring of female mice exposed to varying doses of X-rays *Mutat Res*; **106**: 73–83.

Kirk KM, Lyon MF, 1984. Induction of congenital malformations in the offspring of male mice treated with X-rays at pre-meiotic and post-meiotic stages. *Mutat Res*; **125**: 75–85.

Kline J, Shrout P, Stein Z, Susser M, Warburton D, 1980. Drinking during pregnancy and spontaneous abortion. *Lancet*; **ii**: 176–80.

Kline J, Stein ZA, Susser M, Warburton D, 1977. Smoking: a risk factor for spontaneous abortion. *New Engl J Med*; **297**: 793–6.

Kline J, Levin B, Stein Z, Susser M, Warburton D, 1981. Epidemiologic detection of low dose effects on the developing fetus. *Environ Health Perspec*; **42**: 119–26.

Knoll JH, Chudley AE, Gerrard JW, 1984. Fragile (X) X-linked mental retardation: II Frequency and replication pattern of fragile (X) (q28) in heterozyotes. *Am J Hum Genet*; **36**: 640–5.

Knudsen I, 1986. ed. *Genetic toxicology of the diet.* New York: Alan Liss. (Progress in Clinical and Biological Research 206).

Knudsen I, Hansen EV, Meyer OA, Poulsen E, 1977. A proposed method for the simultaneous detection of germ cell mutations leading to fetal death and of malformations in mammals. *Mutat Res*; **48**: 267–70.

Knuth VA, Hull MGR, Jacobs HS, 1977. Amenorrhoea and loss of weight. *Br J Obstet Gynaecol*; **84**: 801–7.

Kocisova J, Rossner P, Binkova B, Bavorova H, Sram RJ, 1988. Mutagenicity studies on paracetamol in human volunteers: I Cytogenetic analysis of peripheral lymphocytes and lipid peroxidation in plasmas. *Mutat Res*; **209**: 161–5.

Kodama Y, 1982. Cytogenetic and dermatoglyphic studies on severely handicapped patients in an institution. *Acta Med Okayama*; **36**: 383–97.

Koller S, 1983. *Risikofaktoren der Schwangerschaft*. Heidelberg: Springer-Verlag.

Komatsu H, Kakizoe T, Niijima T, Kawichi T, Sugimura T, 1982. Increased sperm abnormalities due to dietary restriction. *Mutat Res*; **93**: 439–46.

Konstantinova B, Bratanova N, 1969. Chromosomal aberrations in patients with ulcerohaemorrhagic colitis. *Digestion*; **2**: 329–37.

Kram D, Schneider EL, 1987. Parental-age effects. Increased frequencies of genetically abnormal offspring. In: Schneider EL, ed. *The genetics of aging*. New York: Plenum Press, 27–49.

Kübler W, Moch KJ, 1975. Zur Deckung des Vitaminbedarfs in der Schwangerschaft. In: Brubacher G, Ritzel G, eds. *Zur Ernährungssituation der schweizerischen Bevölkerung*. Vienna: Hans Huber, 233–41.

Kuhnlein HV, Kuhnlein V, Bell PA, 1983. The effect of short-term dietary modification on human fecal mutagenic activity. *Mutat Res*; **113**: 1–12.

Kuhnlein HV, Levander OA, King JC, Sutherland B, Piskie L, 1981. Dietary selenium and fecal mutagenicity in young men. *Fed Proc*; **40**: 903.

Kummet T, Moon TE, Meyskens FL, 1983. Vitamin A: Evidence for its preventive role in human cancer. *Nutr Cancer*; **5**: 96–106.

Kundsin PB, Ampola M, Streeter S, Neurath, P, 1971. Chromosomal aberrations induced by T strain mycoplasmas. *J Med Genet*; **8**: 181–7.

Kurvink K, Bloomfield CD, Cervenka J, 1978. Sister chromatid exchange in patients with viral disease. *Exp Cell Res*; **113**: 450–3.

Lai CN, Butler MA, Matney TS, 1980. Antimutagenic activities of common vegetables and their chlorophyll content. *Mutat Res*; **77**: 245–50.

Lamson SH, Hook EB, 1980. A simple function for maternal age-specific rates of Down syndrome in the 20-to-49 year age range and its biological implications. *Am J Hum Genet*; **32**: 743–53.

Lang K, 1955. Listeria-Infection als mögliche Ursache früh erworbener Cerebralschäden. *Z Kinderheilk*; **76**: 328.

Langman J, van Faassen F, 1955. Congenital defects in the rat embryo after partial thyroidectomy of the mother animal. *Am J Ophthalmol*; 40: 65–76.

Larson CA, Nyman GE, 1973. Differential fertility in schizophrenia. *Acta Psychiatr Scand*; **49**:272–80.

Lawrie CA, Renwick AG, Sims J, 1985. The urinary excretion of bacterial amino acid metabolites by rats fed saccharin in the diet. *Food Chem Toxicol*; **23**: 445–50.

Lecorché, E. 1885. Du diabète dans ses rapports avec la vie utérine, la menstruation et la grossesse. *Annales de Gynécologie*; **24**: 257–73.

Liang JC, Hsu TC, Henny JE, 1983. Cytogenetic assays for mitotic poisons. *Mutat Res*; **113**: 467–9.

Licznerski G, Lindsten J, 1972. Trisomy 21 in man due to maternal non-disjunction during the first meiotic division. *Hereditas*; **70**: 153–4.

Lindeskog P, Övervik E, Nilsson L, Nord CE, Gustafsson JÅ, 1988. Influence of fried meat and fiber on cytochrome P–450 mediated activity and excretion of mutagens in rats. *Mutat Res*; **204**: 553–63.

Lubs ML, 1981. Mutation rates in severe hemophilia A and Duchenne muscular dystrophy. In: Hook EB, Porter IH, eds. *Population and biological aspects of human mutation*. New York: Academic Press, 91–116.

Lutwak-Mann C, 1964. Observations on progeny of thalidomide-treated male rabbits. *Br Med J*; **ii**: 1090–1.

Lutwak-Mann C, Schmid K, Keberle H, 1967. Thalidomide in rabbit semen. *Nature*; **214**: 1018–20.

Lyon MF, 1981. Sensitivity of various germ-cell stages to environmental mutagens. *Mutat Res*; **87**: 323–45.

Lyon MF, 1985. Measuring mutation in man. *Nature*; **318**: 315–6.

Lyon MF, 1988. Experimental work on induced mutations. *Phil Trans R Soc Lond*; **B 319**: 341–51.

Lyon MF, Renshaw R, 1986. Induction of congenital malformations in the offspring of mutagen treated mice. In: Ramel C, Lambert B, Magnusson J, eds. *Genetic Toxicology of Environmental Chemicals, Part B, Genetic Effects and Applied Mutagenesis*. New York: Liss, 449–58.

Lyon MF, Renshaw R, 1988. Induction of congenital malformation in mice by parental irradiation: transmission to later generations. *Mutat Res*; **198**: 277–83.

Lyon MF, Phillips RJS, Fisher G, 1979. Dose-response curves for radiation induced gene mutations in mouse oocytes and their interpretation. *Mutat Res*; **63**: 161–73.

McKusick VA, 1988. *Mendelian inheritance in Man*. Baltimore: Johns Hopkins University Press. 8th Edition.

McLaren A, 1982. The embryo. In: Austin CR, Short RV, eds. Reproduction in mammals Book 2: Embryonic and fetal development. Cambridge University Press, 1–25.

McLean BK, Rubel A, Nikitovitch-Winer MB, 1977. The differential effects of exposure to tobacco smoke on the secretion of luteinizing hormone and prolactin in the proestrous rat. *Endocrinology*; **100**: 1566–70.

Mandello C, Giorgi R, Nuzzo F, 1984. Chromosomal effects of methotrexate on cultured human lymphocytes. *Mutat Res*; **139**: 67–70.

Mahon R, 1972. Consultations d'un couple avant une grossesse. In: Amiel C, Brettes P, Briard-Guillemot ML et al., *Perinatalité*. Paris: INSERM et Masson, 1–5.

Maine D, McNamara R, 1985. *Birth spacing and child survival*. Columbia University, Center for Population and Family Health.

Mann T, Lutwak-Mann CL, 1981. *Male Reproductive Function and Semen*. Heidelberg: Springer-Verlag.

Martin EC, 1978. Birth intervals and development of nine-year-olds in Singapore. *IPPF Medical Bulletin*; **12**: 1–3.

Martin GM, Sprague CA, Epstein CJ, 1970. Replicative life span of cultivated human cells. *Lab Invest*; **23**: 86–92.

Martin RH, Rademaker A, 1988. The relationship between sperm chromosomal abnormalities and sperm morphology in humans. *Mutat Res*; **207**: 159–64.

Mason KE, 1933. Differences in testes injury and repair after vitamin A deficiency, vitamin E deficiency and inanition. *Am J Anat*; **52**: 153–239.

Maternity Alliance, 1990. *Getting fit for pregnancy* and *Think about a baby? A man's guide to preconception health*. 15 Britannia Street, London WC1X 9JP.

Mathur U, Datta SL, Mathur BBL, 1977. The effect of aminopterin induced folic acid deficiency on spermatogenesis. *Fertil Steril*; **28**: 1356–60.

Mattei JF, Mattei MG, Ayme S, Giraud F, 1982. Contribution of the male to zygotic anomalies. In: Spira A, Jouannet P, eds. *Les facteurs de la fertilité humaine*. Paris INSERM, 171–81.

Mau G, Netter P, 1974. Die Auswirkungen des väterlichen Zigarettenkonsums auf die perinatale Sterblichkeit und die Missbildungshäufigkeit. *Dtsch Med Wochenschr*; **99**: 1113–8.

Meisner LF, Inhorn SL, 1972. Chemically induced chromosome changes in human cells. *Acta Cytol*; **16**: 41–7.

Menzies RC, Crossen PE, Fitzgerald PH, Gunz FW, 1966. Cytogenetic and cytochemical studies on marrow cells in B12 and folate deficiency. *Blood*; **28**: 581–94.

Menzinger G, Gallucca F, Andreani D, 1966. Klinefelter's syndrome and diabetes mellitus. *Lancet*; **i**: 747.

Mikamo K, 1982. Meiotic chromosomal radiosensitivity in primary oocytes of the Chinese hamster. *Cytogenet Cell Genet*; **33**: 88–94.

Mikamo K, Hamaguchi H, 1975. Chromosomal disorder caused by preovulatory overripeness of oocytes. In: Blandau RJ, ed. *Aging gametes – their biology and pathology*. Basel: S. Karger, AG, 72–97.

Mikamo K, Kamiguchi Y, 1983. Primary incidences of spontaneous chromosomal anomalies and their origins and causal mechanisms in the Chinese hamster. *Mutat Res*; **108**: 265–78.

Millar MJ, Elcoate PV, Mawson CA, 1957. Sex hormone control of the zinc content of the prostate. *Can J Biochem Physiol*; **35**: 865–8.

Milunsky A, 1969. Glucose intolerance in the parents of children with Down's syndrome. *Amer J Ment Defic*; **74**: 475–8.

Mitranond V, Sobhon P, Tosukhowong P, Chindaduangrat W, 1979. Cytological changes in the testes of vitamin-A-deficient rats. *Acta Anat*; **103**: 159–68.

Montreal Diet Dispensary. Annual Reports, 2182 Lincoln Ave, Montréal, H3H 1JE, Quebec, Canada.

Morita K, Hara M, Kada T, 1978. Studies on natural desmutagens; screening for vegetable and fruit factors active in inactivation of mutagenic pyrolysis products from amino acids. *Agric Biol Chem*; **42**: 1235–8.

Morley D, Lovel H, 1986. *My name is today*. London: Macmillan for UNICEF.

Morrow DA, 1980a. Nutrition and fertility. *Modern Veterinary Practice*; **61**: 499–503.

Morrow DA, 1980b. The role of nutrition in dairy cattle reproduction. In: Morrow DA, ed. *Current Therapy in Theriogenology*. Philadelphia: Saunders, 449–55.

Mortimer D, Leslie EE, Kelly RW, Templeton AA, 1982a. Morphological selection of human spermatozoa *in vivo* and *in vitro*. *J Reprod Fertil*; **64**: 391–9.

Mortimer D, Templeton AA, Lenton EA, Coleman RA, 1982b. Semen analysis parameters of a population of suspected infertile men. In: Spira A, Jouannet P, eds. *Les facteurs de la fertilité humaine*. Paris: INSERM, 91–5.

Moser HW, 1985. Biologic factors of development. In: Freeman, JM, ed. Prenatal and perinatal factors associated with brain disorders. Washington DC: US Department of Health and Human Services; NIH Publication no 85–1149.

Müller-Tyl P, Riss P, Janisch H, Fischl F, Deutinger J, 1984. Physiology of the ovarian follicle. *Arch Androl*; **12**: 149–56.

Mulley JC, Sutherland GR, 1983. Protease inhibitor (PI) phenotype of individuals with chromosomal fragile sites. *Ann Genet (Paris)*; **26**: 143–6.

Muñoz G, Malavé IB, 1979. Influence of dietary protein restriction on ovulation, fertilization rates and pre-implantation embryonic development in mice. *J Exp Zool*; **210**: 253–8.

Murdoch JL, Walker BA, Hall JG, Abbey H, Smith KK, McKusick VA, 1970. Achondroplasia – a genetic and statistical survey. *Ann Hum Genet*; 33: 227–44.

Myers CR, 1938. An application of the control group method to the problem of the etiology of mongolism. *Proc Amer Assoc Mental Defic*; **62**: 142.

Nagao T, 1987. Frequency of congenital defects and dominant lethals in the offspring of male mice treated with methylnitrosourea. *Mutat Res*; **177**: 171–8.

Navarrete VN, Torres IH, Rivera IR, Shor VP, Garcia PM, 1967. Maternal carbohydrate disorder and congenital malformations. *Diabetes*; **16**: 127–30.

Nelson KB, Deutschberger J, 1970. Head size at one year as a predicator of four-year IQ. *Dev Med Child Neurol*; **12**: 487–95.

Nelson ME, Fisher EC, Catsos PD, Meredith CN, Turksoy RN, Evans WJ, 1986. Diet and bone status in amenorrheic runners. *Am J Clin Nutr*; **43**: 910–6.

Nelson MM, Evans HM, 1949. Pteroylglutamic acid and reproduction in the rat. *J Nutr*; **38**: 11–24.

Nelson MM, Evans HM, 1954. Maintenance of pregnancy in the absence of dietary protein with estrone and progesterone. *Endocrinology*; **55**: 543–9.

Nelson MM, Evans HM, 1955. Relation of thiamine to reproduction in the rat. *J Nutr*; **55**: 151–63.

Nelson MM, Lyons WR, Evans HM, 1951. Maintenance of pregnancy in pyridoxine-deficient rats when injected with estrone and progesterone. *Endocrinology*; **48**: 726–32.

Nelson MM, Lyons WR, Evans HM, 1953. Comparison of ovarian and pituitary hormones for maintenance of pregnancy in pyridoxine-deficient rats. *Endocrinology*; **52**: 585–9.

Newberne PM, Suphakarn V, 1983. Nutrition and cancer; a review with emphasis on the role of vitamins C and E and selenium. *Nutr Cancer*; **5**: 107–19.

Newmark HL, Mergens WJ, 1981. Blocking nitrosamine formation using ascorbic acid and alpha-tocopherol. In: Bruce WR, Correa P, Lipkin SR, Tannenbaum SR, Wilkins TD, eds. *Gastrointestinal cancer, endogenous factors: Banbury Report 7.* Cold Spring Harbor: Banbury, 285–304.

Nielsen J, 1966. Diabetes mellitus in parents with Klinefelter's syndrome, *Lancet*; **i**: 1376.

Nielsen J, 1972a. Diabetes mellitus in patients with aneuploid chromosome aberrations and in their parents. *Humangenetik*; **16**: 165–70.

Nielsen J, 1972b. Immunological aberrations in patients with aneuploid chromosome abnormalities and in their parents. *Humangenetik*; **16**: 171–6.

Nillius SJ, 1978. Epidemiology and endocrinology of weight-loss related amenorrhoea. In: Jacobs HS, Beard RW, eds. *Advances in gynaecological endocrinology.* London: Royal College of Obstetricians and Gynaecologists, 118–30.

Niswander KR, Gordon M, 1972. *The women and their pregnancies.* Washington: US Department of Health, Education & Welfare.

Niswander KR, Jackson EC, 1974. Physical characteristics of the gravida and their association with birthweight and perinatal death. *Am J Obstet Gynecol*; **119**: 306–13.

Nomura T, 1975. Transmission of tumors and malformations to the next generation of mice subsequent to urethane treatment. *Cancer Res*; **35**: 264–6.

Nomura T, 1978. Changed urethane and radiation response of the mouse germ cell to tumour induction. In: Severi L, Knudsen AG, Franmen JF, eds. *Tumours of Early Life in Man and Animals.* Perugia: Grafica di Silvi, 873–91.

Nomura T, 1982. Parental exposure to X rays and chemicals induces heritable tumours and anomalies in mice. *Nature*; **296**: 575–7.

Oakberg EF, 1979. Timing of oocyte maturation in the mouse and its relevance to radiation-induced cell killing and mutational sensitivity. *Mutat Res*; **59**: 39–48.

Obe G, 1984. ed. *Mutations in Man.* Berlin Springer-Verlag.

Omori M, Chytil F, 1982. Mechanism of vitamin A action. *J Biol Chem*; **257**: 14370–4.

Omran AR, Standley CC, 1976. *Family formation patterns and health.* Geneva: World Health Organization.

Ong T, Whong WZ, Stewart J, Brockman HE, 1986. Chlorophyllin: a potent antimutagen against environmental and dietary complex mixtures. *Mutat Res*; **173**: 111–5.

Ong T, Whong WZ, Stewart JD, Brockman HE, 1989. Comparative antimutagenicity of 5 compounds against 5 mutagenic complex mixtures in salmonella typhimurium strain TA 98. *Mutat Res*; **222**: 19–25.

OPCS: Office of Population Censuses and Surveys, 1983. *Congenital malformation statistics, series MB3 no. 1.* London: HMSO.

OPCS: Office of Population Censuses and Surveys, 1987. *Infant and perinatal mortality 1985: birthweight, series OH3 87/1.* London: HMSO.

OPCS: Office of Population Censuses and Surveys, 1988. *Congenital malformation statistics, series MB3 No 2..* London: HMSO.

Pandy VK, Parmeshwasan M, Soman SD, 1983. Concentrations of morphologically normal, motile spermatozoa: Mg, Ca and Zn in the semen of infertile men. *Science Total Environment*; **27**: 49–52.

Papiernik E, 1978. La grossesse et les déficiences intellectuelles de l'enfant. *Arch Fr Péd*; **35**: x–xiv.

Parry Jones A, Murray W, 1958. The heights and weights of educationally subnormal children. *Lancet*; **ii**: 905.

Penrose LS, 1955. Parental age and mutation. *Lancet*; **ii**: 312.

Peterson RN, Freund M, 1975. The inhibition of the motility of human spermatozoa by various pharmacologic agents. *Biol Reprod*; **13**: 552–6.

Phillips LS, Vassilopoulou-Sellin R, 1979. Nutritional regulation of somatomedin. *Am J Clin Nutr*; **32**: 1082–96.

Pierson H, 1936. Experimentale Erzeugung von Uterusgechwülsten bei Kaninchen durch Prolan. *Z Krebsforschung*; **45**: 1–27.

Poland BJ, Miller JR, Harris M, Livingston J, 1981. Spontaneous abortion: a study of 1961 women and their conceptuses. *Acta Obstet Gynecol Scand (Suppl. 102)*.

Pond WG, Wagner WC, Dunn JA, Walker EF, 1968. Reproduction and early postnatal growth of progeny in swine fed a protein-free diet during gestation. *J Nutr*; **94**: 309–16.

Population Reports, 1983. *Infertility and sexually transmitted disease*. Series L No. 4, Baltimore: Johns Hopkins University Press.

Potier de Courcy G, 1966. Caractère globaux des métabolismes nucléique et protéique chez le foetus de rat carencé en acide pantothénique. *Arch Sci Physiol*; **20**: 43–63.

Potier de Courcy G, Bujoli J, 1981. Effects of diet with or without folic acid, and with and without methionine, on fetus development, folate stores and folic acid dependent enzyme activities in the rat. *Biol Neonate*; **39**: 132–40.

Potier de Courcy G, Desmettre M, Miguet S, 1970. Effets de la carence en riboflavine sur quelques éléments minéraux des tissus foeto-maternels du rat. *Arch Sci Physiol*; **24**: 183–95.

Potier de Courcy G, Terroine T, 1968. Conséquences chez le rat de la carence en riboflavine sur la composition globale de certains tissus maternels et foetaux. *Arch Sci Physiol*; **22**: 329–55.

Powers AC, Eisenbarth GS, 1985. Autoimmunity to islet cells in diabetes mellitus. *Annu Rev Med*; **36**: 533–44.

Reidy JA, Zhou X, Chen ATL, 1983. Folic acid and chromosome breakage. *Mutat Res*; **122**: 217–21.

Ritzel G, 1975. Evaluation von Ernährungserhebungen im Rahmen der Basler Studie III. In: Brubacher G, Ritzel G, eds. *Zur Ernährungssituation der schweizerischen Bevölkerung*. Bern: Verlag Hans Huber, 57–82.

Ross ML, Pike RL, 1956. The relationship of vitamin B6 to protein metabolism during pregnancy in the rat. *J Nutr*; **58**: 251–67.

Rush D, 1986. Nutrition in the preparation for pregnancy. In: Chamberlain G, Lumley J, eds. *Prepregnancy care: a manual for practice*. Chichester: John Wiley, 113–39.

Rush D, Alvir JM, Kenny DA, Johnson SS, Horwitz DG, 1988. Historical study of pregnancy outcomes. In: The National WIC Evaluation. *Am J Clin Nutr*; **48**: 412–28.

Russell LB, 1956. Dominant lethals induced at a highly sensitive stage in mouse oogenesis. *Anat Rec*; **125**: 647–8.

Russell LB, Russell WL, 1956. The sensitivity of different stages in oogensis to the radiation induction of dominant lethals and other changes in the mouse. In: Mitchell JS, Holmes BE, Smith CC, eds. *Progress in Radiobiology*. Edinburgh: Oliver & Boyd, 187–92.

Russell WL 1977. Mutation frequencies in female mice and the estimation of genetic hazards of radiation in women. *Proc Natl Acad Sci*; **74**: 3523–7.

Russell WL, 1986. Positive genetic hazard predictions from short-term tests have proved false for results in mammalian spermatogonia with all environmental chemicals so far tested. In: Ramel B, Lambert B, Magnusson J, eds. *Genetic toxicology of environmental chemicals. part B: Genetic effects and applied mutagenesis*. New York: Alan Liss, 67–74. (Progress in Clinical and Biological Research 209)

Russell WL, Hunsicker PR, 1983. Extreme sensitivity of one particular germ-cell stage in male mice to induction of specific-locus mutation by methylnitrosourea. *Environ Mutagen*; **3**: 498.

Sanborn CF, Martin BJ, Wagner WW, 1982. Is athletic amenorrhoea specific to runners? *Am J Obstet Gynecol*; **143**: 859–61.

Sanger R, Tippett P, Gavin J, Teesdale P, Daniels GL, 1977. Xg groups and sex chromosome abnormalities in people of northern European ancestry. *J Med Genet*; **14**: 210–1.

Sauberlich HE, Dowdy RP, Skala JH, 1977. *Laboratory tests for the assessment of nutritional status*. Cleveland: CRC Press.

Schempp W, Krone W, 1979. Deficiency of arginine and lysine causes increase in frequency of sister chromatid exchanges. *Hum Genet*; **51**: 315–8.

Schmauch G, 1899. Ueber endoglobuläre Körperchen in den Erythrocyten der Katze. *Virchows Arch*; **156**: 201–44.

Schneider EL, 1978. Cytogenetics of aging. In: Schneider EL, ed. *The genetics of aging.* New York: Plenum Press, 27–49.

Schneider EL, 1980. Aneuploidy and ageing. In: *Conference on Structural Pathology and the Biology of Ageing.* Freiburg: Zentrallaboratorium für Mutagenitätsprüfung, 221–34.

Schorah CJ, 1981. Vitamin C status in population groups. In: Counsell JN, Hornig DH, eds. *Vitamin C (ascorbic acid).* London: Applied Science Publishers, 23–47.

Schroeder TM, 1982. Genetically determined chromosomal instability syndromes. *Cytogenet Cell Genet*; **33**: 119–32.

Schroeder WT, Chao LY, Das DD, *et al.*, 1987. Non-random loss of maternal chromosome 11 alleles in Wilm's tumors. *Am J Hum Genet*; **40**: 413–20.

Schroeder-Kurth TM, Auerbach AD, Obe G, 1989, eds. *Fanconi's Anemia; clinical, cytogenetic and experimental aspects.* Heidelberg: Springer-Verlag.

Scottish Health Service, 1977. *Scottish Health Statistics, 1976.* Edinburgh.

Seeliger HPR, 1961. *Listeriosis.* Basel: S. Karger A.G.

Sharma G, Polasa H, 1978. Cytogenetic effects of influenza virus infection on male germ cells of mice. *Hum Genet*; **45**: 179–87.

Sharp AA, Witts LJ, 1962. Seminal vitamin B12 and sterility. *Lancet*; **ii**: 779.

Sherer GK, Jackson BB, Leroy EC, 1981. Chromosome breakage and sister chromatid exchange frequencies in scleroderma. *Arthritis Rheum*; **24**: 1409–13.

Schimkin MB, Grady HG, 1940. Mammary carcinomas in mice following oral administration. *Z Krebsforsch*; **52**: 158–9.

Sjödin P, Jägerstad M, 1984. A balanced study of ^{14}C labelled 3-H-imidazo [4, 5–f] quinolin-2-amines (IQ and MeIQ) in rats. *Food Chem Toxicol*; **22**: 207–10.

Slater E, Hare EH, Price JS, 1971. Marriage and fertility of psychiatric patients compared with national data. *Soc Biol; 18 (Suppl)*:S60–S73.

Smith CG, 1983. Reproductive toxicity; hypothalamic-pituitary mechanisms. *Am J Ind Med*; **4**: 107–12.

Smith MD, 1962. Seminal vitamin B12 and sterility. *Lancet*; **ii**: 934.

Smith TE, 1960. The Cocos-Keeling Islands: a demographic laboratory. *Population Studies*; **14**: 94–7.

Smithells RW, Nevin NC, Seller MJ *et al.*, 1983. Further experience of vitamin supplementation for prevention of neural tube defect recurrences. *Lancet*; **i**: 1027–31.

Soyka LF, Joffe JM, 1980. Male mediated drug effects on offspring. In: Schwarz RH, Yaffe SJ, eds. *Drug and chemical risks to the fetus and newborn.* New York: Alan Liss, 49–60.

Spätling L, 1987. Die Frühgeburt vor der 34sten Schwangerschaftswoche. *Gynäkologe (Berlin)*; **20**: 4–13.

Spätling L, Spätling G, 1986. Magnesium supplementation in pregnancy: a double-blind study. *Magnesium Bull*; **8**: 252–3.

Spätling L, Spätling G, 1988. Magnesium supplementation in pregnancy: a double-blind study. *Br J Obstet Gynaecol*; **95**: 120–5.

Sperling K, 1984. Frequency and origin of chromosome abnormalities in man. In: Obe G, ed. *Mutations in Man.* Heidelberg: Springer-Verlag, 128–46.

van der Spuy ZM, Steer PJ, McCusker M, Steele SJ, Jacobs HS, 1988. Outcome of pregnancy in underweight women after spontaneous and induced ovulation. *Br Med J*; **296**: 962–5.

Stavric B, 1984. Mutagenic food flavonoids. *Fed Proc*; **43**: 2454–8.

Steel JM, Johnstone FD, Smith AF, Duncan LJP, 1982. Five years' experience of a "prepregnancy" clinic for insulin-dependent diabetics. *Br Med J*; **285**: 353–6.

Stein Z, Susser M, Saenger G, Marolla F, 1975. *Famine and human development.* Oxford University Press.

Steinberg SE, Fonda S, Campbell CL, Hillman RS, 1983. Cellular abnormalities in folate deficiency. *Br J Haematol*; **54**: 605–12.

Stevenson AC, 1978. Effect of twelve folate analogues on human lymphocytes *in vitro*. In: Evans HJ, Lloyd DC, eds. *Mutagen-induced chromosome damage in man.* Edinburgh University Press. 227–38.

Stoll C, Roth MP, Bigel P, 1982. A reexamination of parental age effect on the occurrence of new mutations for achondroplasia. New York: Alan Liss, 419–26. (Progress in Clinical and Biological Research 104)

Stölzner W, 1919. Zur Aetiologie des Mongolismus. *Münch Med Wochenschr*; **66**: 1493–4.

Sugimura T, 1985. Carcinogenicity of mutagenic heterocyclic amines formed during the cooking process. *Mutat Res*; **150**: 33–41.

Sugimura T, Nagao M, 1982. The use of mutagenicity to evaluate carcinogenic hazards in our daily lives. In: Heddle JA, ed. *Mutagenicity: new horizons in genetic toxiocology*. New York, London: Academic Press, 73–88.

Sümbüloglu K, Bertan M, Fisek NH, 1976. In: Omran AR, Standley CC, eds. *Family formation patterns and health*. Geneva: World Health Organization, 191–9.

Sussman A, Leonard JM, 1980. Psoriasis, methotrexate, and oligospermia. *Arch Dermatol*: **116**: 215–7.

Sveriges officiella statistik, 1979. *Allmän hälso och sjukvård 1976*. Stockholm.

Tagami S, Sudo K, 1982. Influence on ovulation and ovulated ova in mice of different dietary protein levels and feeding periods. *Jpn J Zootech Sci*; **53**: 266–71.

Takahara H, Cosentino MJ, Cockett ATK, 1982. Zinc therapy alone or in combination with varicocelectomy to improve the fertility potential of the male *J Androl*; **3**: 37.

Tawn EJ, Cartmell CL, 1989. The effect of smoking on the frequencies of asymmetrical and symmetrical chromosome exchanges in human lymphocytes. *Mutat Res*; **224**: 151–6.

Templeton AC, 1970. Generalized herpes simplex in malnourished children. *J Clin Pathol*; **23**: 24–30.

Terwel L, van der Hoeven JCM, 1985. Antimutagenic activity of some naturally occurring compounds towards cigarette-smoke condensate and benzo [a] pyrene in the salmonella/microsome assay. *Mutat Res*; **152**: 1–4.

Thalhammer O, 1967. *Pränatale Erkrankungen des Menschen*. Stuttgart: Thieme Verlag.

Tharapel AT, Tharapel SA, Bannerman RM, 1985. Recurrent pregnancy losses and parental chromosome abnormalities: a review *Br J Obstet Gynaecol*; **92**: 899–914.

Thompson S, Lopez B, Wong K-H, *et al.*, 1982. A prospective study of chlamydia and mycoplasma infections during pregnancy. In: Mårdh PA, Moller B, Paavonen J, eds. Chlamydia trachomitis in genital and related infections. *Scand J Infect Dis* (suppl 32); 155–8.

Thompson LH, Tucker JD, Stewart SA, *et al.*, 1987. Genotoxicity of compounds from cooked beef in repair-deficient CHO cells versus salmonella mutagenicity *Mutagenesis*; **2**: 483–7.

Timmermans L, 1974. Influence of antibiotics on spermatogenesis. *J Urol*; **112**: 348–9.

Togucida J, Ishizaki K, Sasaki MS, *et al.*, 1989. Preferential mutation of paternally derived RB gene as the initial event in sporadic osteosarcoma. *Nature*; **338**: 156–8.

Tomaszewski L, Zmudzka B, Nadworny J, 1963. Seminal vitamin B12 and sterility. *Lancet*; **i**: 170.

Torkelson TR, Sadek SE, Rowe UK, *et al.*, 1961. Toxicologic investigation of 1,2 dibromo-3-chloropropane. *Toxicol Appl Pharmacol;* **3**: 545–9.

Toth A, Lesser ML, Brooks C, Labriola D, 1980. Subsequent pregnancies among 161 couples treated for T-mycoplasma genital-tract infection. *New Eng J Med*; **308**: 505–7.

Trasler JM, Hales BF, Robaire B, 1985. Paternal cyclophosphamide treatment of rats causes fetal loss and malformations without affecting male fertility. *Nature*: **316**: 144–6.

Trémolières, J, 1977. *Nutrition, physiologie, comportement alimentaire*. Paris: Dunod.

Tsuboi T, Endo S, 1977. Incidence of seizures and EEG abnormalities among offspring of epileptic patients. *Hum Genet*; **36**: 173–89.

Tsuchida WS, Uchida JA, 1974. Chromosome aberrations in spermatocytes and oocytes of mice irradiated prenatally. *Mutat Res*; **22**: 277–80.

Tunbridge WMG, Evered DC, Hall R, *et al.*, 1977. The spectrum of thyroid disease in a community: The Whickham survey. *Clin Endocrinol (Oxf)*; **7**: 481–93.

Unglaub-Leisten I, Stickl H, Frick E, Angstwurm H, Ring J, 1975. Chromosomenuntersuchungen an peripheren Lymphozyten bei Patienten mit multipler Sklerose. *Dtsch Med Wochenschr*; **100**: 2028–34.

US Centers for Disease Control, 1989. Contribution of birth defects to infant mortality, US 1986. *Morbidity & Mortality Weekly Report*; **38**: No. 37.

US Department of Labor Occupational Safety and Health Administration, 1978. Occupational exposure to lead: final standard. Federal Register; 43 No 220: 52952–53014.

US National Academy of Sciences, 1980. *Recommended dietary allowances 9th ed.* Washington DC.

US National Center for Health Statistics, 1972. *A study of infant mortality from linked records.* DHEW Publication No. (HMS) 72–1055, Rockville, Maryland.

US National Center for Health Statistics, 1978. *Characteristics of Births, United States 1973-75* DHEW Publication No. (PHS) 78–1908, Rockville, Maryland.

US National Center for Health Statistics, 1979. *Dietary Intake Source Data, United States 1971-74* DHEW Publication No. (PHS) 79–1221, Hyattsville, Maryland.

US National Center for Health Statistics, 1987. Prevalence of known diabetes among Black Americans. Advance Data No. 130 DHEW Pub. No. (PHS) 87–1250, Hyattsville, Maryland.

US National Research Council, 1982. *Diet, nutrition, and cancer.* Washington DC: National Academy Press.

US Surgeon-General, 1980. *The health consequences of smoking for women.* Washington DC: US Department of Health and Human Services.

Vigersky RA, Loriaux DL, 1977. Anorexia nervosa as a model of hypothalamic dysfunction. In: Vigersky RA, ed. *Anorexia nervosa* New York: Raven Press, 109–21.

Vogel F, 1984. Gene or point mutations. In Obe G, ed. *Mutations in Man*, Heidelberg: Springer-Verlag, 101–27.

Wais S, Salvati E, 1966. Klinefelter's syndrome and diabetes mellitus. *Lancet*; **i**: 747.

Warkany J, 1971. *Congenital malformations.* New York: Year Book Medical Publishers.

Warkany J, Schraffenberger E, 1944. Congenital malformations induced in rats by maternal nutritional deficiency. *J Nutr*, **27**: 477–84.

Warren MP, 1977. Weight loss and responsiveness to LH-RH. In: Vigersky RA, ed. *Anorexia nervosa.* New York: Raven Press. 189–98.

Watanabe G, 1979. Environmental determinants of birth defects prevalence. *Contributions to Epidemiology and Biostatistics*; **1**: 91–100. Basel: S Karger, AG.

Watson AA, 1962. Seminal vitamin B12 and sterility. *Lancet*; **ii**: 644.

Watteville H, Jürgens R, Pfalz H, 1954. Einfluss von Vitaminmangel auf Fruchtbarkeit, Schwangerschaft und Nachkommen. *Schweiz Med Wochenschr*; **84**: 875–82.

Wauben–Penris PJJ, van Buul-Offers SC, 1982. Meiotic disjunction in male Snell dwarf mice. *J Hered*; **73**: 365–9.

Weitberg AB, 1989. Effect of nicotinic acid supplementation *in vivo* on oxygen radical-induced genetic damage in human lymphocytes. *Mutat Res*; **216**: 197–201.

Werbach MR, 1989. *Nutritional influences on illness.* Wellingborough: Thorson.

Whorton MD, Milby TH, 1980. Recovery of testicular function among DBCP workers, *J Occup Med*; **22**: 177–9.

Wiesner PJ, Parra WC, 1982. Sexually transmitted diseases: meeting the 1990 objectives – a challenge for the 1980s. *Public Health Rep*; **97**: 409–16.

Westöm L, 1980. Incidence, prevalence, and trends of acute pelvic inflammatory disease and its consequences in industrialized countries. *Am J Obstet Gynecol*; **121**: 707–13.

Weström L, Mårdh PA, 1983. Chlamydial salpingitis. *Br Med Bull*; **39**: 145–50.

Whincup PH, Cook DG, Shaper AG, 1989. Early influences on blood pressure; a study of children aged 5–7 years. *Br Med J*; **299**: 587–91.

Wilkins JF, Kilgour RJ, 1982. Production responses in selenium supplemented sheep in northern New South Wales. *Aust J Exp Agric Anim Husbandry*; **22**: 18–28.

Williams DL, Hagen AA, Runyan JW, 1971. Chromosome alterations produced in germ cells of dogs by progesterone. *J Lab Clin Med*; **77**: 417–29.

Winter RM, 1987. Population genetics implications of the premutation hypothesis for the generation of the fragile-X mental retardation gene. *Hum Genet*; **75**: 269–71.

Wolner-Hanssen P, Mårdh PA, 1984. *In vitro* tests of the adherence of *chlamydia trachomatis* to human spermatozoa. *Fertil Steril*; **42**: 102–7.

World Health Organization, 1981. *World Health Statistics*, Geneva.

Wynn AHA, Crawford MA, Doyle Wendy, Wynn SW, 1991. Nutrition of women in anticipation of pregnancy. *Nutr Health*; **7**: 69–88.

Wynn M, Wynn A, 1979. *Prevention of handicap and the health of women*. London: Routledge.

Wynn M, Wynn A, 1981a. The importance of nutrition around the time of conception in the prevention of handicap. *Hum Nutr: Appl Nutr*; **1**: 12–18.

Wynn M, Wynn A, 1981b. *The prevention of handicap of early pregnancy origin: some evidence for the value of good health before conception*. London: Foundation for Education & Research in Childbearing.

Wynn M, Wynn A, 1981c. Historical associations of congenital malformations. *Int J Environ Stud*; **71**: 7–12.

Wynn M, Wynn A, 1982. *Lead and Human Reproduction*. London: Campaign for Lead-free Air.

Wynn M, Wynn A, 1987. Nutrition before conception and the outcome of pregnancy. *Nutr Health*. **5**: 31–43.

Wynn M, Wynn A, 1987. *Preconception hazards of alcohol, smoking and cannabis: Symposium City University London*. Maidenhead: Wyeth.

Wynn M, Wynn A, 1988a. Health around conception: the health of the mother. *Postgraduate Doctor*; **11**: 305–16. Barker Publications, 539 London Road, Middlesex TW7 4DA.

Wynn M, Wynn A, 1988b. Magnesium and other nutrient deficiencies as possible causes of hypertension and low birthweight. *Nutr Health*. **6**: 69–88.

Wynn M, Wynn A, 1989. Health around conception: health of the father. *Postgraduate Doctor*; **12**: 592–606. Barker Publications, 539 London Road, Middlesex TW7 4DA.

Wyrobek AJ, 1982. Methods for evaluating the influence of chemicals on human male fertility. In: Spira A, Jouannet P, eds. *Les facteurs de la fertilité humaine*. Paris: INSERM, 295–310.

Wyrobek AJ, Bruce WR, 1975. Chemical induction of sperm abnormalities in mice. *Proc Natl Acad Sci*; **72**: 4425–29.

Wyrobek AJ, Gordon AL, Burkhart JG, *et al.*, 1983. An evaluation of human sperm as indicator of chemically induced alterations of spermatogenic function. *Mutat Res*; **115**: 73–148.

Yamamoto M, Endo A, Watanabe G, Ingalls TH, 1971. Chromosomal aneuploidies and polyploidies in embryos of diabetic mice. *Arch Environ Health*; **22**: 468–75.

Yamamoto M, Ito T, Watanabe M, Watanabe G, 1982. Causes of chromosomal anomalies suggested by cytogenetic epidemiology of induced abortions. *Hum Genet*; **60**: 360–4.

Yano K, 1979. Effect of vegetable juices and milk on alkylating activity of N-methyl-N-nitrosourea. *J Agric Food Chem*; **27**: 456–8.

Yerushalmy J, Bierman JM, Kemp DH, Connor A, French FE, 1956. Longitudianal studies of pregnancy on the island of Kauai, territory of Hawaii. *Am J Obstet Gynecol*; **71**: 80–96.

Zacharias JF, Jenkins JH, Marion JP, 1984. The incidence of neural tube defects in the fetus and neonate of insulin-dependent diabetic women. *Am J Obstet Gynecol*; **150**: 797.

Zellers JE, Gautieri RF, 1977. Evaluation of teratogenic potential of codeine sulphate in CF–1 mice. *J Pharmacol Sci*; **66**: 1727–31.

Zuppinger K, Engel E, Forbes AP, Mantooth L, Claffey J, 1967. Klinefelter's syndrome, a clinical and cytogenetic study in twenty-four cases. *Acta Endocrinol (Copenh)*; **113**: 5–48.

Index